Workouts
for Women

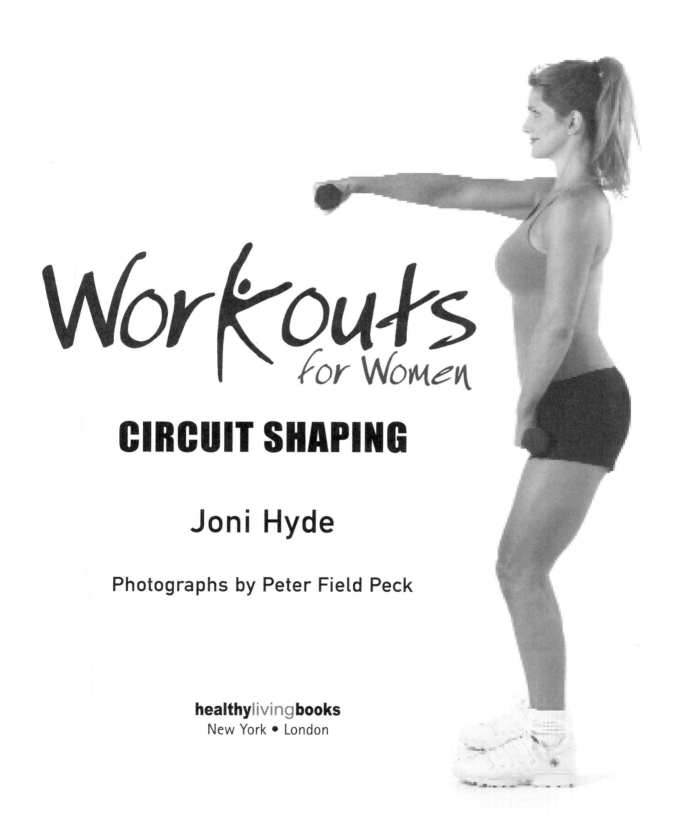

Workouts for Women

CIRCUIT SHAPING

Joni Hyde

Photographs by Peter Field Peck

healthyliving**books**
New York • London

Healthy Living Books
Hatherleigh Press
5-22 46th Avenue, Suite 200
Long Island City, NY 11101

www.healthylivingbooks.com

Hyde, Joni.
  Workouts for women / by Joni Hyde.
      p. cm.
  ISBN 1-57826-183-X
 1. Exercise for women. 2. Physical fitness for women. I. Title.
  GV482.H93 2004
  613.7'045--dc22

                                        2004021932

Information included in this book is for your general knowledge only and is not intended as a substitute for the advice or care of medical professionals. Please consult your physician or other healthcare professional before starting any new physical fitness program.

All Healthy Living Books titles are available for special promotions and premiums. For more information, please contact the manager of our Special Sales department at 800-528-2550.

ISBN 1-57826-183-X

Interior Design by Calvin Lyte and Deborah Miller
Cover Design by Deborah Miller
Exercise Photos by Peter Field Peck

Printed in Canada
10 9 8 7 6 5 4 3 2 1

Table of Contents

Welcome to

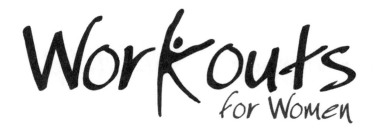

Y ou've taken the first step toward empowering yourself as a woman... by making fitness a part of your lifestyle.

I have so much enthusiasm for fitness because of the way it's changed my life and the lives of so many women that I've worked with. I've created this program to provide a unique way for more women like you to enjoy the benefits of personal training.

I love the long-term benefits of working out and I've seen the results through the years working with my clients. They're setting a positive example for their children... and I know first hand how great it feels when my little girl watches me exercise. Other women have told me they notice that the quality of their relationships has improved, and they notice an immediate increase in their self-esteem.

It's also been proven that women who work out on a consistent basis dramatically reduce their levels of stress, and their bodies are healthier. Taking care of ourselves is so important in keeping our energy levels high and in keeping us youthful no matter what age we are.

To me, taking care of ourselves is not something that we do when all else fails, but it's a way of creating a balanced self that gives us the confidence to shine as empowered women.

The great thing about this program is that you don't have to be locked in to a trainer's schedule or recreate your own schedule when you feel you can't add one more thing to your lifestyle. You work out when it's convenient for you.

Circuit Training–style gyms for women are extremely popular throughout the nation as well as internationally. These gyms offer focused exercises that are

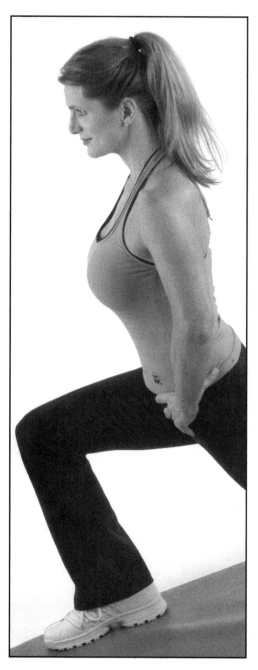

structured into a fast and convenient way to perform a total-body aerobic and strength-training workout. I've designed these ten 12-minute routines so now you can experience Circuit Training in the comfort and convenience of your own home. These workouts are time-efficient and easy to follow, and they really work.

These routines offer great flexibility. They're ideal for a quick lunchtime or late afternoon workout in the middle of a hectic day. When you want a full workout, you can perform a circuit two, three, or four times giving you up to a 48-minute workout.

Remember... you start where you are, and the key to seeing the benefits of working out is simply giving it time to show the results. With consistency and a healthy diet, within just 2 to 3 weeks you will notice a difference and start to hear those compliments from family and friends.

Congratulations on taking the biggest step...making the decision to begin.

Stay fit and healthy.
Joni Hyde, your personal trainer

Visit us on the web at
www.WorkoutsForWomen.com

Welcome to
Workouts for Women

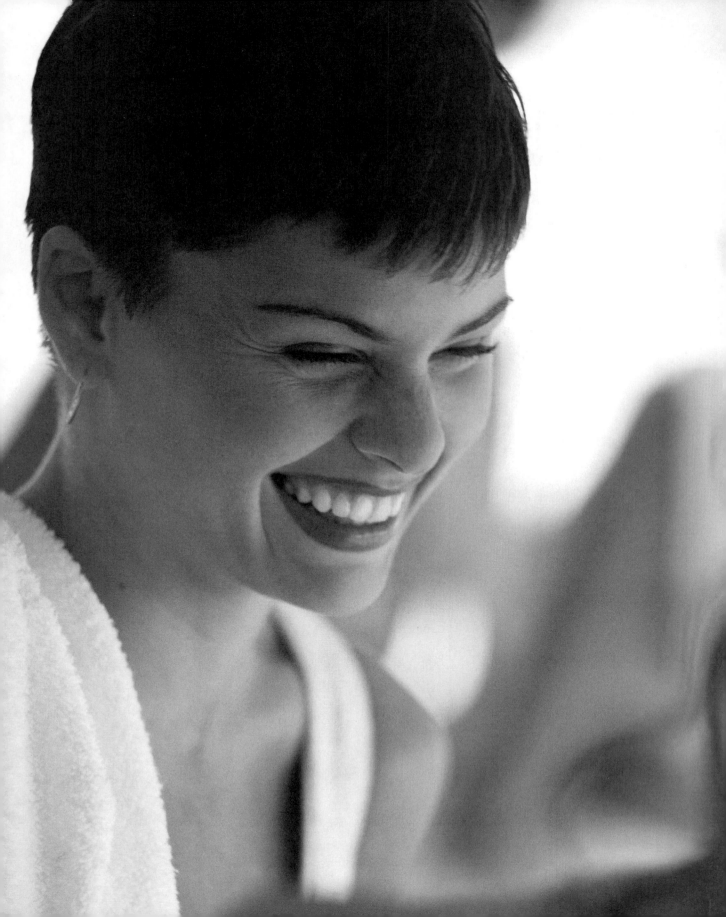

Part
1

Getting Started

The Power of Circuit Training

We Are Different

It's perfectly clear that the ideal woman's body is very different from the ideal man's body. Men and women gain, store, and burn fat differently, and since women naturally have much less muscle mass then men, women have a much harder time keeping fat under control. Because of these obvious differences, doesn't it make sense that a woman should have an exercise program that is specifically designed for her goals?

Many women hit the gym with a vengeance and follow a program that is the same as their boyfriend's or husband's. Since women have much less testosterone than men, the potential to get as big and strong as our male counterparts is not there; however some women can see a substantial increase in their muscle size if they train like a man.

We are all predisposed to respond to exercise in a certain way, simply because of our genetics and body type. Many women's bodies respond to weight training by getting larger when lifting very heavy weights. When it comes to strength training, you can still count on one of the old rules: To get bigger use heavier weights and fewer repetitions (6 to 8), and allow rest time for muscle recovery to gain size. To lose weight and inches and to tighten and tone, train with lighter weights, more repetitions (10 to 15) and higher frequency (3 to 6 days a week).

Why is it so much harder for women to lose weight than it is for men? Women naturally have more body fat than men. That is something that is out of our control. This means that, as women, we have more fat mass as opposed to muscle mass. Fat is metabolically less active than muscle. So, in other words, men have the advantage of having more lean muscle tissue, which is a more metabolically active tissue. But this is not to say that there isn't anything that we can do about it. Eating a healthy high-fiber diet and incorporating an exercise routine into your lifestyle that includes both cardiovascular activity and strength training is key to shedding fat and pounds.

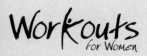

What Is Circuit Training?

Circuit Training is one of the most versatile methods of exercising. If you are committed to burning fat, shaping up, and improving your overall health and quality of life, then circuit training is for you. This type of training provides a one-stop total body exercise session, combining aerobic and strength training into a highly efficient workout.

This type of program is ideal for women who are ready to lose fat, reduce the appearance of cellulite, firm up, and tackle those problem areas... the hips, thighs, butt, abdomen, and the backs of the arms.

Circuit Training is a method of exercise whereby you move from one exercise to the next in a quick-paced progression, performing one set of each exercise. By rotating exercises, you give muscle groups a rest period before they are worked again, resulting in better fatigue management.

The variety of exercises in each circuit as well as the multiple routines included in this book will keep your mind interested and will keep your body stimulated, resulting in ongoing improvements in your physique.

Spot Removal Works Only for the Laundry

Women often focus on exercising a particular body part which is hidden by fatty tissue in an effort to "burn away" the localized fat and expose toned muscles. However, spot removal only works in the laundry, not on your body. There is simply no such thing as localized fat loss. Fat is lost evenly throughout the body. No amount of crunches will reveal a well-toned abdomen if your body is storing extra body fat.

KEY FEATURES OF CIRCUIT TRAINING

- Circuit Training is flexible. If you are short on time you can do one complete total-body workout in about 10 minutes. If you have time for a more challenging workout, you can do up to four Circuits, completing up to a 45-minute workout.
- Whatever your level of fitness, whether you're an athlete or merely a beginner, you can work at a pace that is comfortable for you.
- The quick-paced activity involved in Circuit Training is an excellent fat burner.
- Circuit Training is psychologically rewarding and challenging, offering loads of variety.
- Circuit Training can be done at home or the gym.
- The benefits of Circuit Training can be summed up in a few words: "Maximum results in the minimum amount of time."

LIFTING WEIGHTS TO LOSE WEIGHT

Lifting weights improves your metabolism in two ways. The activity itself burns calories, and the muscles you build increase your body's use of calories even at rest. One lb. of muscle burns about 45 calories a day, while one lb. of fat only burns about 4 calories. The more muscle you pack onto your body, the faster your metabolism and the sleeker you will look!

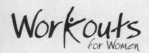

If you're struggling with a "trouble spot," here's the deal. To remove the fat from your trouble spots you need to increase your overall percentage of lean muscle mass and combine that with a healthy diet.

The Three-in-One Advantage of Circuit Training

Circuit Training will keep you moving from one exercise to the next in a quick pace... keeping your heart rate up and keeping your body burning calories while you are exercising.

At the same time you will be gaining lean muscle mass. This is so significant because in our mid-twenties we begin to lose muscle mass as part of the normal aging process. This loss of muscle slows down our metabolism, resulting in the storage of fat. Aerobics-only programs will not counteract this loss of muscle, but as you Circuit Train you will be building lean muscle mass. For each pound of lean muscle mass that you gain, your body will burn up to approximately 45 more calories at rest per day! This in combination with a healthy diet is the key to long term weight control.

Finally, you'll be shaving off inches and sculpting your body into a well-toned feminine physique.

It's Not Your Imagination

If you have not experienced it yourself yet, you've heard other women talk about their metabolism slowing down. Just wait and you will be in that same predicament. With that slowdown comes weight gain even if your eating habits did not change. The good news is, there is a way to reverse these effects, and the answer is not hours upon hours of aerobic activity or trying the newest fad diet. Aerobic activity does nothing to replace or help to maintain muscle mass and fad diets alone will only cause you to lose more muscle mass.

To speed up your metabolism to its original capacity you have to replace the muscle mass that you have lost.

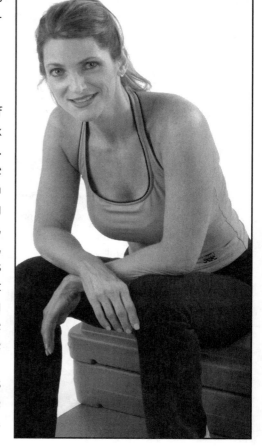

Some women have questioned whether or not they should choose an aerobics only program until they reach their ideal weight, and the answer is NO! Don't wait! You must replace lean muscle mass to increase your metabolism 24/7 and the only way to do that is with strength training.

Increase your metabolism, shape, tone and shave inches in one efficient workout...Circuit Train.

DON'T BE RULED BY THE SCALE

Since muscle weighs more than fat, as you become more fit, the numbers on the scale may lead you to think you are not truly making progress. The scale may not always be the best indicator of how effective your workouts are. Check out your progress with a measuring tape and by the way your clothes fit.

The Power of Circuit Training

Planning Your Workouts

Fitting In Fitness

Finding the time to exercise can be tough, but if you make a plan and schedule your workout time in advance you'll be much more likely to get it done. Simply put, if you fail to plan, you plan to fail.

With kids, jobs, school, and all the other responsibilities of home and family, where does exercise fit in? Here are some ideas on finding the time to exercise and making it happen.

1. Make exercise a priority. If you're serious about getting fit you will find the time to exercise.

2. Write down your typical daily schedule. Once it is on paper you may see blocks of time that can be used better so you can fit exercise in.

3. Work out the same time every day. If you make it a daily routine, it becomes your special time to take care of yourself.

4. Wake up 30 minutes earlier and work out in the morning if you can. There is less chance that something won't crowd exercise out in the morning than later in the day.

5. Turn off the TV. The average adult spends 16 hours a week watching TV. Cut out a few hours and you'll have more time to fit in exercise and other chores.

The Right Time to Exercise

There is no concrete research which has proven that either morning or evening workouts provide superior metabolic benefits. However, morning and evening workouts do each have their own benefits.

One thing is for sure: One time does not fit all when it comes to exercise. The important thing is that you exercise consistently. Choose a time that is convenient and enjoyable for you.

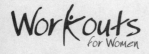

Benefits of Early Workouts

1. Exercising early is the only way to ensure that other chores that come up during the day won't keep you from doing your workout.

2. Surveys report that most individuals who regularly exercised did so in the morning. So if you're a morning exerciser you'll be more likely to stick with it.

3. Research has shown that exercise increases mental sharpness for 4 to 10 hours post-exercise.

4. Many women who exercise in the morning say they have more energy the rest of the day.

5. Some people claim that morning exercise regulates their appetite for the day, making them less hungry.

Benefits of Afternoon or Evening Workouts

1. Previous research concluded that a late workout would disrupt sleep. New research has reported that this assumption is not valid. Researchers say that you can exercise up to 30 minutes before bedtime without disrupting sleep patterns. In fact, it may help you fall asleep faster.

2. Afternoon is the best time to exercise for optimal workout performance quality.

3. Muscles are warm and more flexible in the afternoon.

4. Exercise is a good stress reliever after a long day.

5. Strength is at its peak in the afternoon.

In the end, the best time for you to exercise is whatever works well for you. If your schedule permits, I always suggest exercising in the morning. Energy levels are higher in the morning than they are later in the day, so you'll probably get a better workout. Also, exercising further increases your level of energy, making you feel better all day long. Morning workouts also save you the chore of having to re-do make up and hair, which you would have to do if you worked out at lunch time or after work. So, wake up, work out, shower, and go! You'll have the whole day ahead of you.

Planning Your Workouts

7

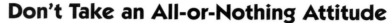

Don't Take an All-or-Nothing Attitude

When the going gets tough, remember some exercise is better than none. When life throws unexpected curveballs into your schedule, scale back on your workouts but don't quit. Exercise should not be an all-or-nothing type deal.

Take care of yourself and maintain your regular workouts—you will feel better and have more energy. Even if you have to cut your workouts back, you will be far better off than if you did no exercise at all.

Also, don't feel guilty when you have to miss a workout or two. Negative feelings only hinder motivation. Believe in yourself! Think of exercise in the right perspective. Exercise is an investment in yourself.

How Often Can I Circuit Train?

If you are trying to lose weight and inches as you re-shape and tone your body, Circuit Training can offer you the best results and a decrease in size when the muscles are not allowed to recover fully, so training as many as 4 to 6 days a week is advised for maximum decrease in inches.

The lower weight–higher repetition approach used in Circuit Training is safe to do on consecutive days. Once you've attained your goals, a program of performing your routine two to three times a week will maintain strength and your new physique.

Always take at least one or two days off each week or you will risk burnout.

Planning the Workout for Your Fitness Level

There are 10 different Circuit workouts included in this book. Each Circuit is appropriate for either a beginner or intermediate exerciser. To increase or decrease the difficulty of your workout, simply increase or decrease the amount of weight you are using and/or complete more or fewer rotations of Circuits.

If you are a new exerciser, start out with just one Circuit each day that you work out. In other words, choose a Circuit and complete one set of all 10 exercises in that Circuit. Once your fitness level increases and completing just one Circuit rotation is no longer challenging, then add a second Circuit rotation into your workout. For maximum results, work up to four Circuit rotations each time that you work out. Each Circuit should take 8 to 12 minutes to complete. Four rotations of a Circuit should take approximately 45 to 60 minutes, including a 5- to 10-minute stretch at the end.

During your workout you should move quickly from one exercise to the next, one Circuit to the next without taking a break, except for water.

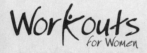

STRETCHING FOR RESULTS

Flexibility is the ability to move a joint throughout its range of motion. Maintaining flexibility is necessary for optimal performance. A body that is flexible is less prone to injury and to low back pain. Studies have shown that stretching may also improve circulation to joints and may actually help decelerate joint degenerative processes.

Stretching at the end of your workout may be the most efficient way to produce permanent gains in flexibility since the muscles and ligament temperatures are slightly elevated. Here are some key points to remember when stretching:

1. Slowly and gradually lengthen the muscle in a controlled manner to the point of slight discomfort.
2. Hold the position for 15 to 30 seconds.
3. Refrain from quick jerky motions or bouncing, which can result in sprains.
4. Proper alignment is critical in achieving maximum benefits. When joints are correctly moved through their full range of motion, flexibility can increase by as much as 50% in women of all ages.

Proper alignment when stretching is critical in achieving maximum benefits. To view video/audio demonstrations of stretches for the major muscles groups, please visit us on the web at http://www.WorkoutsForWomen.com/stretch.asp

Getting the Most Out of Your "Circuit Shaping" Workout

Each Circuit includes 10 exercises. The first exercise always involves the large muscles of the lower body and is primarily intended to increase your heart rate, which warms up the muscles in preparation for the exercises that follow. Make sure that you perform the first exercise of each Circuit at a safe but moderately vigorous pace.

The next nine exercises are lower-body and upper-body strength and endurance exercises. You will complete 12 to 15 repetitions of each exercise. The last exercise in each Circuit is targeted toward the abdomen, torso, and/or back. To train for shape and weight loss, take no rest periods between exercises except for a drink of water.

Equipment Needs
To complete the workouts you'll need the following items:

A Step
There are several different types of steps. I prefer the molded step, because it's in one piece and easy to maneuver, but the other type of step with risers to adjust the height will work as well.

SUBSTITUTIONS: Use any steps around your home.

SCHEDULE WORKOUT APPOINTMENTS
If you schedule your workouts in advance and write them down on your calendar, you're more likely to get it done then if you just work out when you find the time. Remember, you're important and making fitness a priority will keep you going strong.

MAKE IT COUNT

Make each workout count! Push yourself, but not to the point that you're in pain. Just remember, exercise should not be easy, but should be performed at moderate to high intensity depending on your fitness level. If your body is not challenged you won't see any changes.

DUMBBELLS

The typical range is from 2 to 12 lbs. Since some muscle groups are stronger than others, it will be necessary to have several sets of dumbbells to keep the various muscle groups challenged.

When choosing your weights, it's better to start out light. You can always increase, but starting too heavy puts you at risk of injury.

SUBSTITUTIONS: Use canned food or plastic jugs filled with water.

ANKLE WEIGHTS

There are several type of ankle weights on the market. I prefer the adjustable type, which offers the flexibility of using 1 to 10 pounds per leg.

SUBSTITUTIONS: Ankle weights are not necessary, but help to provide extra resistance. For many women, using their own body weight provides enough resistance.

A CHAIR

This should be a sturdy, firm, seated chair that does not slide on the flooring surface that you are working on.

A MAT OR CUSHIONED FLOOR

For your convenience, we offer a variety of equipment in our fitness store at www.WorkoutsForWomen.com.

How To Choose the Right Amount of Weight

"One size fits all" weight recommendations do not offer you the custom program necessary to give you a safe and effective workout, so rather than tell you what weight to use, as your personal trainer, I'll teach YOU how to choose the right amount of weight for you.

The first exercise in each Circuit is a "heart raiser" lasting for 2 minutes. Following the heart raiser are nine total body strength exercises. The idea is to move at a steady pace from one exercise to the next keeping your heart rate elevated, while burning fat and building lean muscle and endurance.

You will be asked to perform 12 to 15 repetitions of each exercise, unless instructed otherwise. The right amount of weight for you will allow you to perform 12 to 15 repetitions of each exercise with the last few repetitions being challenging. If you can do more than 15 repetitions, then you need to slightly increase the weight that you are using. If you can't make it to even 12 repetitions, then you're using too much and you'll need to choose a lighter weight.

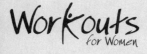

It may take a few times to find the right weight for each exercise, so when you do, write it down so you'll remember for next time. As you continue to work out consistently, your strength and self-esteem will increase. Your body will change and improve... one step at a time.

SHORT CIRCUITS
Don't have a solid hour in a day to spend on exercise? Split up your workouts into two 20 to 30 minute segments. You'll still gain the same benefits as if you had performed one longer workout.

PREVENTING INJURY

Even with the most careful execution, injuries during exercise can occur. The most common injuries are related to tendons and ligaments. A combination of rest, ice, compression and elevation is recommended as a remedy. If pain persists for more than 2 or 3 days, you should consult with your health care provider. Also, seek immediate care if there is any loss of joint motion, swelling, and sharp or severe pain.

Here is a injury regimen called RICE that every exerciser should know.

Rest. Do not use an injured knee, ankle, shoulder, etc. Rest promotes healing.

Ice. Apply ice to a new injury as soon as possible for about 30 minutes. Cold shrinks torn blood vessels and helps to stop internal bleeding. Re-apply the ice three to fives times. After about 72 hours after an injury, apply heat appropriately.

Compression. Wrap the injury firmly but not tightly. This will keep swelling down and reduce motion on the injury.

Elevation. Raise the injured area above heart level if you can. Gravity drains fluid, which will minimize swelling and pain.

Motivate Me!

Need a few words of wisdom to get your fitness program in high gear? First, start slowly. Don't overdo it when you are just beginning your program or just getting back into exercise after taking an extended break.

It's important that you make the commitment to take total responsibility for your physical and emotional health. Make your workout one of your top priorities for each day by making regular exercise appointments and keeping them. Plan ahead but take it one week at a time. Planning out your exercise program on a long-term basis can be a little overwhelming. Create a short-term exercise schedule that you can re-evaluate often.

At times it can be difficult to stay motivated about exercise while juggling work, chores, home, kids, and hobbies. We all have too many responsibilities and too little time. The key is to focus on the benefits that you stand to gain from exercise and make it a priority.

Planning Your Workouts

The motivational process is changing and ongoing. Here are a few practical tips to help keep you focused on your achievements and accountable to yourself.

1. Build on your small successes. Start with small goals. Revel in the small accomplishments. They add up to great things.

2. Be realistic about your goals. It doesn't take a few weeks to get flabby or become overweight, so don't expect to see results over night.

3. Track your progress. Take your measurements so you'll be able to evaluate how your body is changing. Take a photo of yourself now so you'll have visual validation of the changes in your body over time.

4. Focus on why you are doing this. Exercise is an investment in yourself. Don't focus on what you are giving up to become fit, focus on what you are gaining.

5. Use the power of visualization daily. Visualize yourself completing a great work-out and focus on how great you'll feel knowing you got the job done. Visualize yourself reaching your goals.

6. Know your limits and give your body adequate fuel. Fatigue, insomnia, irritability, and an elevated resting heart rate are signs of overdoing it or not getting proper nutrition!

7. Reward yourself when you obtain your goals.

8. Keep a workout log and a food journal. Track your progress by taking your measurements every 6 to 8 weeks. (See Appendix I and II for examples and blank forms.)

Little Steps Toward Big Goals

Most of the women who succeed at reaching and maintaining their fitness goals and living a healthy lifestyle have one major factor in common. They set goals for themselves and write them down.

Your goals should be very specific, and they should be measurable, attainable, and realistic. Unrealistic goals simply set you up for disappointment, and goals that are vague, unrealistic, and impossible to measure can leave you wondering whether or not you are making any progress, which can lead to a decrease in motivation.

Have you thought about what your goals are? If not, do so! Write them down and map out a timeline of when you want to meet your goals with checkpoints for rewards along the way. Rewards are great incentives. Give yourself a treat for

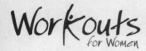

making all your workout appointments for the week: manicures and pedicures, a massage, a long bubble bath are all great treats.

If you are trying to lose weight, be realistic and aim to lose 1 to 2 pounds per week. Weight loss that exceeds 2 pounds per week is not healthy and can slow down your metabolism and put you at risk of losing vital muscle tissue. But don't be ruled by the scale. Since muscle weighs more than fat, as you get fit, the numbers on the scale may lead you to think you are not truly losing. In addition to the scale, track your progress by the way you feel, with a measuring tape and by the fit of your clothes.

Get Ready... Get Set...

Women of all ages are taking advantage of the benefits that lifting weights can give to them. Studies have shown that women who lift weights have a reduced risk of osteoporosis and increase their lean muscle mass. This increase in muscle mass increases the body's ability to burn calories, even at rest!

Weight training plays no favorites when it comes to age. From the young woman trying to reshape her body to the mature woman whose goal is to stay strong, vibrant, and healthy, everyone can benefit.

An exercise program that combines cardiovascular activity and strength training together is the most time-efficient way to exercise. As more women realize that proper strength training will produce a leaner, healthier, stronger body without bulky muscles, they are incorporating strength training into their overall workout routines and are loving the results!

Get Fit Now!

Before you begin your workout, be prepared. Have your water bottle close by, your favorite music on and all of your equipment in place so you can move quickly from one exercise to the next. The time it takes to put on your ankle weights, have a drink of water or get into position for the next exercise is all the rest you should give yourself until you're finished, unless of course you experience any warning signs (dizziness, shortness of breath, etc.) If so, stop immediately.

Now it's time to get moving and create a leaner, shapelier, and stronger body. There is no better time than the present to shape up. Empower yourself as a woman and make fitness a part of your lifestyle!

Planning Your Workouts

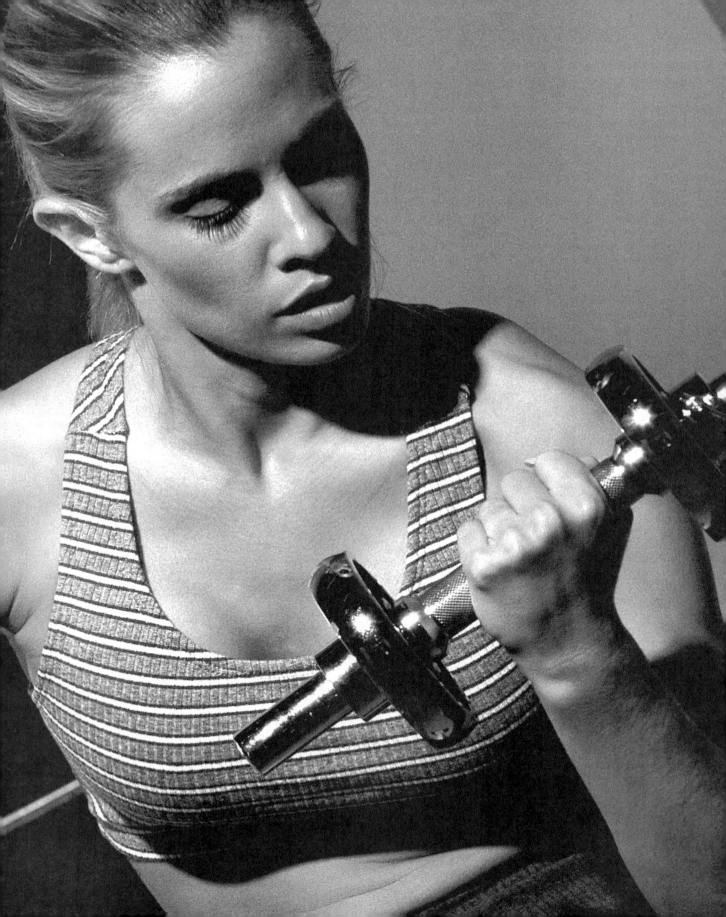

Part
2

The Circuits

ONE

EQUIPMENT
Dumbbells
Ankle Weights
Chair

CIRCUIT

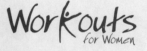

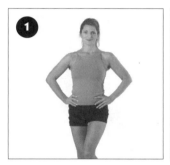

Wide-Step Touches   **PG 17**

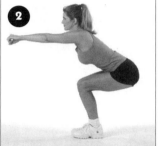

Narrow Squats   **PG 18**

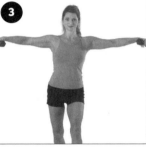

Straight Arm Laterals   **PG 19**

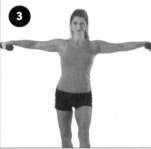

Knee-Up Crunches   **PG 26**

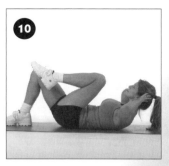

Half Up Bicep Curls   **PG 20**

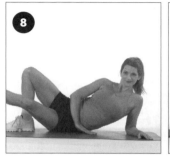

Wide Grip Push-Ups   **PG 25**

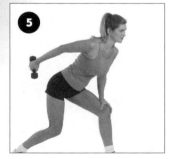

Triceps Lift   **PG 21**

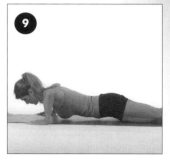

Inner Thigh Pull-In   **PG 24**

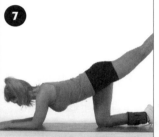

Mule Kick   **PG 23**

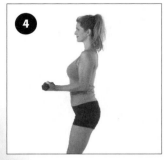

Seated Bent-over Rear Flies   **PG 22**

Wide-Step Touches

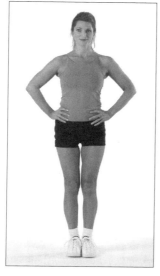 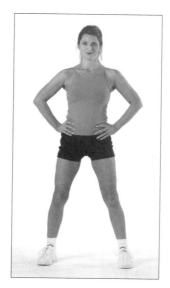

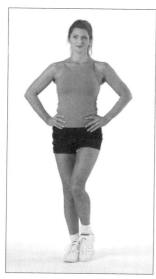 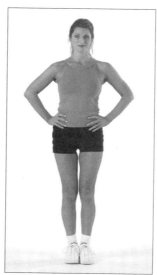

BODY PART WORKED
Cardiovascular System

SET UP
Stand tall with shoulders back, chest high, and abdomen held in tight with hands on your hips.

TIPS FROM JONI
Adding in arm movements will increase your heart rate and the exercise intensity.

Exercise Technique

1. Bend knees slightly and take a step out to the side with one leg, then bring the other leg over to meet with the first leg, tapping the toes onto the floor.

2. Repeat the same motion on the other side.

REPEAT FROM SIDE TO SIDE AT A MODERATE PACE FOR AT LEAST 2 MINUTES.

Circuit One

SET UP

Start standing tall with feet and knees together, abdominal muscles held in tight, shoulders back, chest high, and toes pointed straight ahead.

TIPS FROM JONI

Be sure not to allow your knees to extend past your toes as you lower down or you will be placing too much stress on the knees.

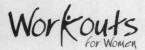

Narrow Squats

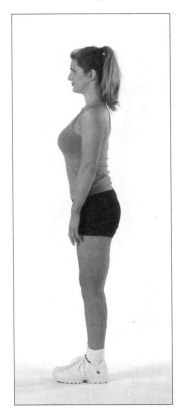 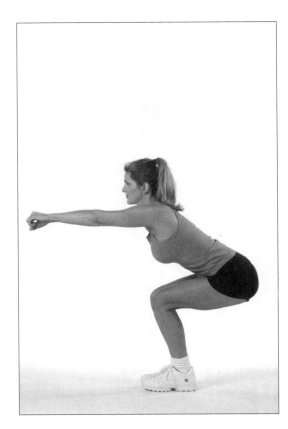

Exercise Technique

1. Bend at the knees and reach back with your buttocks as if you were sitting onto a chair behind you.

2. Stop when your hips are knee level. Do not drop any lower.

3. Exhale as you press yourself back up to standing position with most of your weight pressing up through your heels.

4. Contract the buttocks at the top of the move as you stand back up.

REPEAT 15 TIMES.

Straight Arm Laterals

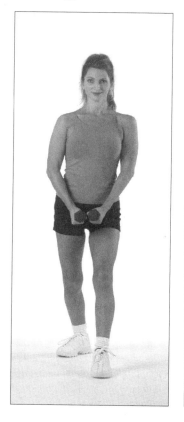 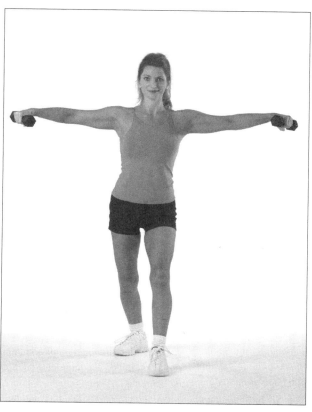

SET UP

Stand tall with feet
together and knees slightly bent with shoulders
back, chest high, and
abdomen held in tight.
Hold a dumbbell in each
hand with arms hanging
down in front of your
body with palms facing in
toward each other.

TIPS FROM JONI

At the top of the move
check for proper form,
being sure that hands and
elbows are at the same
height and that wrists are
straight.

Exercise Technique

1. Exhale as you lift both arms up and out to the sides.

2. Control the resistance as you lower your arms back down to starting position.

REPEAT 15 TIMES.

Circuit One

SET UP

Stand tall with shoulders back, chest high, and abdomen held in tight. Place arms down at your sides, holding a dumbbell in each hand with the palms of your hands facing forward.

TIPS FROM JONI

Be sure not to rock your body as you lift the weight, which will cause you to use momentum rather than your arm muscles.

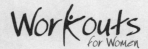

Half-Up Biceps Curls

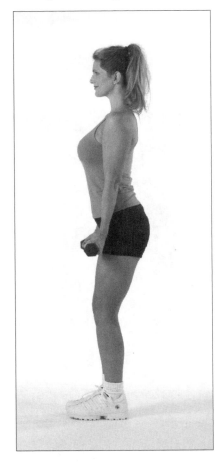 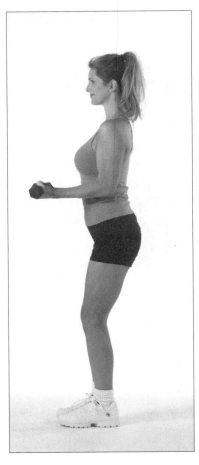

Exercise Technique

1. Keeping your elbows stationary, exhale as you bend arms at the elbows lifting your forearms halfway up, stopping when they are parallel to the floor.

2. In a controlled manner, lower your arms back down to start position.

REPEAT 15 TIMES.

Triceps Lift

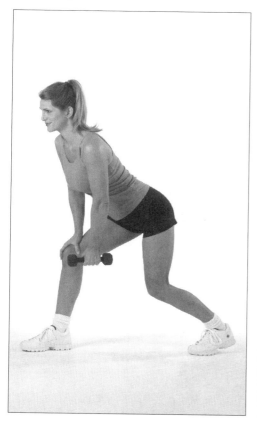 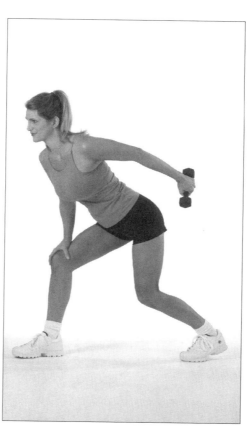

SET UP

Begin this exercise in a semi-lunge position, standing with one leg forward and one back. Both knees should be pointing straight ahead and abdominal muscles should be held in tight. Lean forward, bending at the hip, and rest the forward hand on your forward thigh to support your body. Hold a dumbbell in the other hand and allow that arm to extend straight down.

TIPS FROM JONI

Be sure not to swing the working arm and concentrate on using the muscles in the back of your arm to lift the weight up.

Exercise Technique

1. Exhale as you extend the arm straight back lifting the weight to shoulder height feeling the tension in the back of the arm.

2. Lower the arm back to start in a controlled manner.

REPEAT 15 TIMES ON ONE SIDE THEN ON THE OTHER SIDE.

Circuit One

BODY PART WORKED

Upper Back (Trapezius)

SET UP

Hold a dumbbell in each hand and sit on the edge of a chair. Bend forward at the hips and hold your abdomen in tight. Rest your chest on the thighs with your arms hanging at your sides, palms facing in toward each other.

TIPS FROM JONI

Keep your back and neck in a straight line through-out the move.

Workouts for Women

22

Seated Bent-over Rear Flies

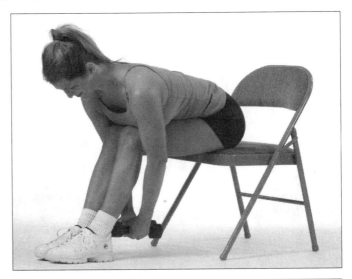

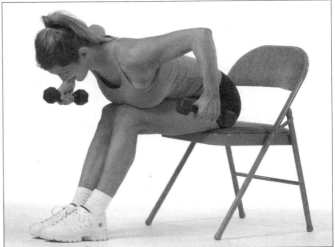

Exercise Technique

1. Exhale as you bend your arms at the elbows, pulling your hands up toward the rib cage, squeezing your shoulder blades together at the top of the move.

2. Reverse the move and lower your arms back to start in a controlled manner.

REPEAT 15 TIMES.

Mule Kick

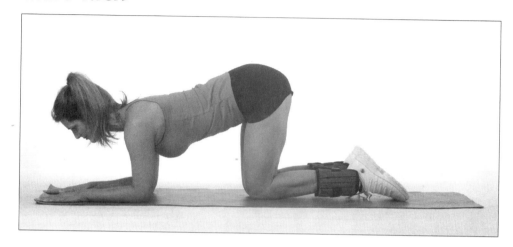

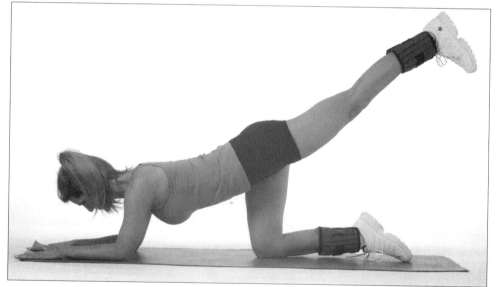

BODY PART WORKED
Buttocks (Gluteal)

SET UP
With ankle weights around each leg, get down on the floor on your knees and forearms with abdomen held in tight.

TIPS FROM JONI
Keep your neck in a relaxed position. Keep both hips square to the floor during the entire movement.

Exercise Technique

1. With your foot flexed, exhale as you kick up and out with one leg, squeezing the buttocks at the top of the motion when your leg is extended.

2. Bend your leg at the knee pulling it back into start position, without resting your knee on the floor.

REPEAT 15 TIMES ON ONE SIDE THEN 15 ON THE OTHER.

Circuit One

SET UP
Lie down on your side
with your bottom leg
extended. Bend the top
leg and place your foot
flat on the floor behind
the bottom leg. Shift your
body weight onto the hip
of your extended leg and
prop your upper body up
with the corresponding
forearm.

TIPS FROM JONI
Keep the foot flexed and
heel pointing upward on
the working leg to keep
the movement focused on
working the inner thigh
muscle.

Workouts
for Women

Inner Thigh Pull-In

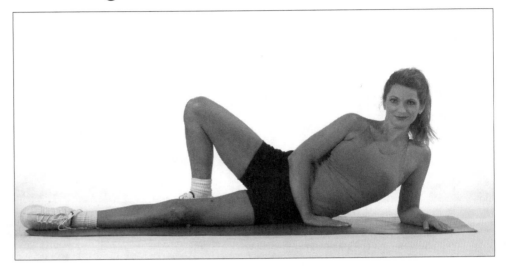

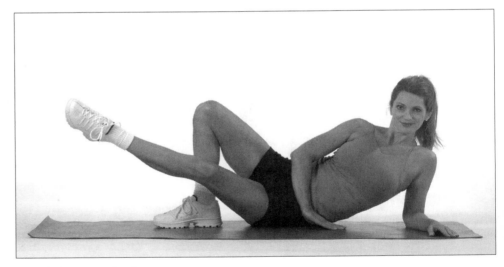

Exercise Technique

1. With your extended foot flexed and heel rotated upward, exhale as you lift
   your leg upward as you simultaneously bend the knee and pull the foot in
   toward you.

2. Extend your leg back out to start again, without resting the leg on the floor.

REPEAT 15 TIMES.

Wide Grip Push-Ups

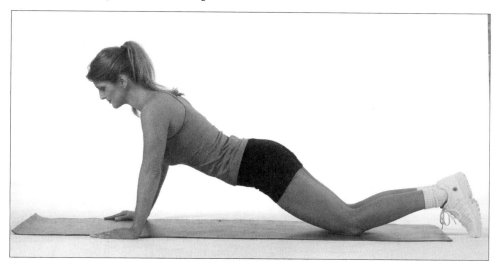

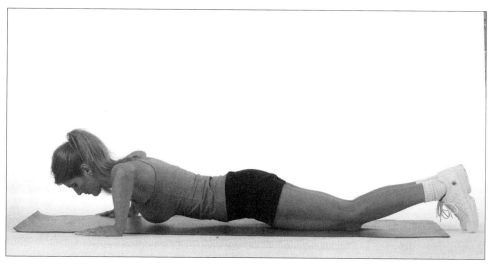

Exercise Technique

1. Bend your elbows and lower your chest. Stop one fist distance from the floor.

2. Exhale as you push your body back up to start again.

REPEAT 15 TIMES.

BODY PART WORKED
Chest (Pectoral)

SET UP
Get down on your hands and knees with hands placed outside shoulder width, fingers facing forward, and knees extended back as far as comfortable. Hold your abdominal muscles in tight.

TIPS FROM JONI
Keep elbows soft (slightly bent) as you extend back up to start position. Keep abdominal muscles tight and your neck in line with your spine at all times. To decrease the difficulty of the move, bring your hands and knees in closer together.

Circuit One

Upper and Lower Abdomen (Rectus Abdominis)

SET UP

Lie flat on your back with your knees bent, heels close to your body, and pelvis tilted slightly upward to help flatten your back. Place your fingertips lightly against the back of your head.

TIPS FROM JONI

Focus on moving your rib cage toward your hip bone as you lift up. Keep your elbows back and out of sight. Keep your chin one fist distance off your chest.

Workouts for Women

Knee-Up Crunches

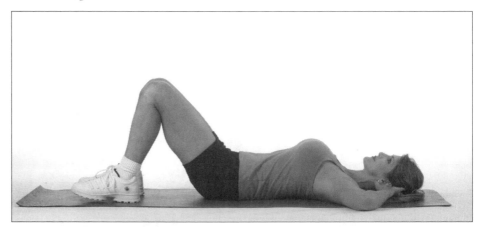

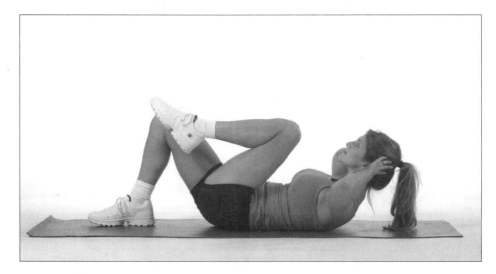

Exercise Technique

1. Exhale as you lift your shoulder blades up and forward while simultaneously bringing one knee up and in toward your chest.

2. Lower your leg back down to start and repeat on the other side without resting your head on the floor.

ALTERNATE FROM SIDE TO SIDE FOR A TOTAL OF 20 TO 30 TIMES.

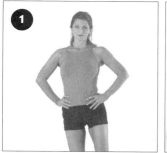

Peg Leg on Step   **PG 28**

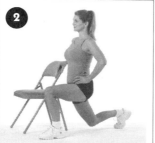

Stationary Lunge   **PG 29**

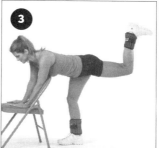

Standing Bent-Leg Curl   **PG 30**

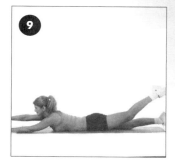

Pulse-up Crunches   **PG 37**

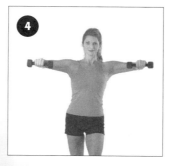

Shoulder Rotators   **PG 31**

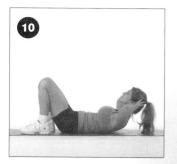

Superwoman   **PG 36**

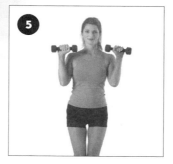

Reverse Biceps Curls   **PG 32**

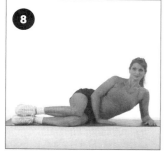

Bent Outer Thigh   **PG 35**

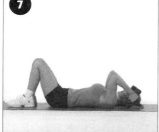

Lying Triceps Extension   **PG 34**

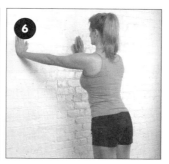

Wide Wall Push-Ups   **PG 33**

TWO

EQUIPMENT
Step
Dumbbells
Ankle Weights
Chair

CIRCUIT

Circuit Two

BODY PART WORKED

Cardiovascular System

SET UP

Stand with one foot in the center of the step and the other foot on the floor. Pull shoulders back, hold chest high, and pull abdominal muscles in tight.

TIPS FROM JONI

Be sure not to lock your knees when stepping up. Go at your own pace.

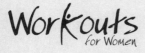

Peg Leg on Step

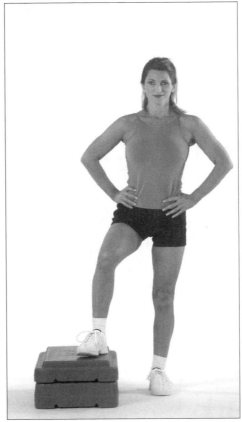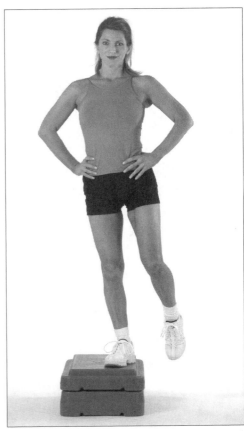

Exercise Technique

1. Press up with the heel of the foot that is on the step. This will straighten the knee and lift the other foot off the floor.

2. Return the foot to the floor, landing on the ball of the foot, while the foot on the step simultaneously lifts up off the step.

REPEAT THIS STEPPING MOTION ON THE SAME SIDE FOR ABOUT ONE MINUTE THEN WALK AROUND TO THE OTHER SIDE OF THE STEP AND REPEAT FOR ANOTHER MINUTE.

Stationary Lunge

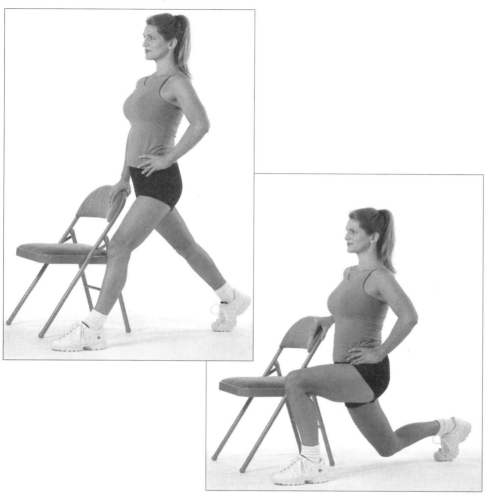

BODY PART WORKED
Thighs (Adductor, Abductor, Quadriceps)

SET UP
Kneel down, then step one leg forward with the heel directly below the ankle. Now stand up. Your legs should be shoulder-width apart and the heel of the rear foot should be up. Pull your shoulders back hold your chest out, and hold your abdomen in tight. Hold onto a chair for balance if you need to.

TIPS FROM JONI
Be careful not to lock your knees as you return to start. As you lower down, be sure that your front knee stays directly over your ankle and does not move over past your toes.

Exercise Technique
1. Bend both knees and lower your hips toward the floor, stopping before your back knee touches the ground.

2. Exhale as you straighten your knees and press yourself up with the heel of your forward foot and the toes of your back foot, lifting your body straight up to start.

REPEAT 10 TIMES ON EACH SIDE.

Circuit Two

Workouts
for Women

30

Standing Bent-Leg Curl

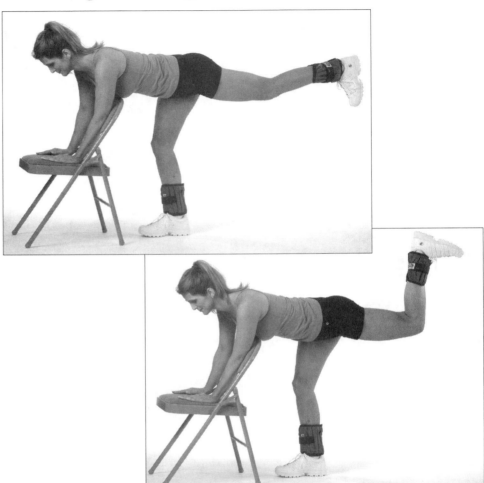

Exercise Technique

1. Exhale as you bend the extended leg at the knee, pulling your heel up toward your buttocks.

2. Extend the leg back out in a controlled manner, being sure not to let the leg drop.

REPEAT 15 TIMES ON ONE SIDE, THEN 15 TIMES ON THE OTHER.

Shoulder Rotators

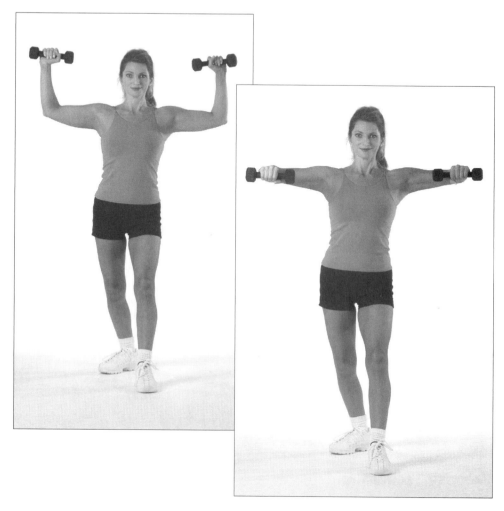

BODY PART WORKED
Shoulders (External Shoulder Rotator)

SET UP
Stand tall with dumbbells in hands and abdomen held in tight. Bend arms at the elbows up to a goal-post position with palms facing forward.

TIPS FROM JONI
Elbows should remain at shoulder height through-out the entire move.

Exercise Technique

1. Rotate forearms forward bringing palms facing downward, stopping when forearms are parallel to the floor.

2. Exhale and keep upper arms stationary as you return back to start.

REPEAT 15 TIMES.

Circuit Two

SET UP
Stand tall with shoulders back, chest high, and abdomen held in tight. Place arms directly in front of your thighs, holding dumbbells in each hand with palms of your hands facing in toward you.

TIPS FROM JONI
Be sure that your elbows remain stationary and close to your body throughout the entire move.

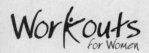

Reverse Biceps Curls

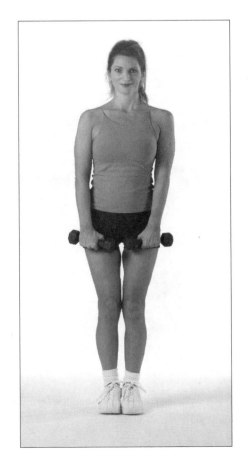
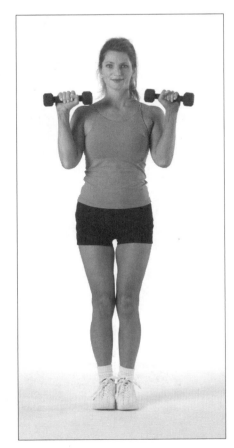

Exercise Technique

1. Exhale and bend at the elbows, bringing your hands up toward your shoulders with palms facing forward at the top of the move.

2. In a controlled manner, lower your arms back down to start position.

REPEAT 15 TIMES.

Wide Wall Push-Ups

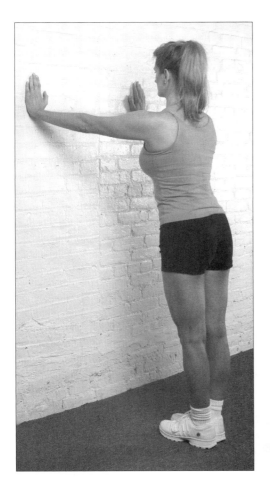
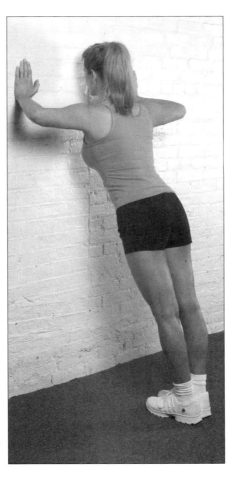

SET UP

Stand about a foot and a half away facing a wall. Place your hands flat on the wall just outside shoulder width, at shoulder height. Hold abdominal muscles in tight.

TIPS FROM JONI

Adjust the difficulty of this move by moving your feet further away from the wall for an increased challenge, or closer to the wall to reduce the challenge.

Exercise Technique

1. Bend your elbows until your chest is a few inches from the wall.

2. Exhale as you push with your hands back to start position.

REPEAT 15 TIMES.

SET UP

Lie flat on your back with your knees bent and feet flat on the floor. With dumbbells in both hands, extend your arms straight up from the shoulders with palms facing in towards each other.

TIPS FROM JONI

Forearms should remain extended straight up from the shoulders throughout the entire exercise, which will keep the exercise focused and effective for the back of the arm.

Lying Triceps Extension

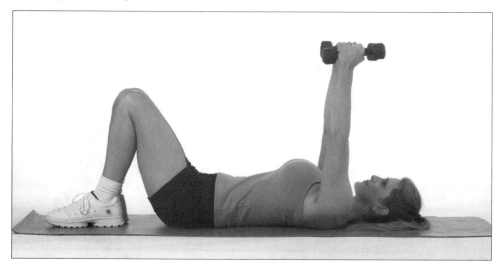

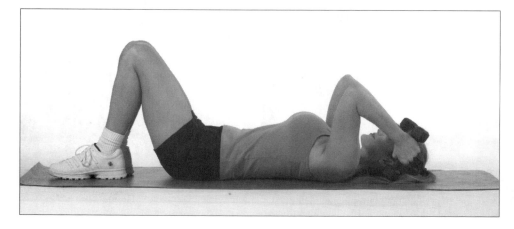

Exercise Technique

1   Keeping your upper arms stationary, bend at the elbows and lower your hands toward your shoulders.

2   Exhale as you extend your arms back up to start, being careful not to lock your elbows at the top of the move.

REPEAT 15 TIMES.

Bent Outer Thigh

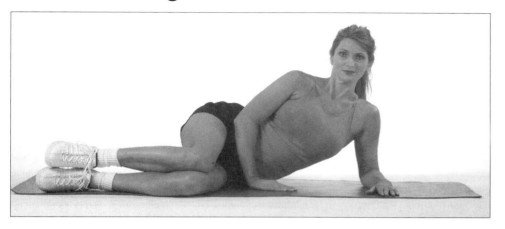

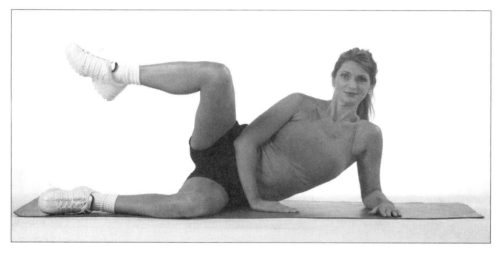

Exercise Technique

1. Exhale as you lift the top leg as high as you can, keeping your knee bent and motionless.

2. Control the leg as you lower back to start without resting the leg down.

REPEAT 15 TIMES ON ONE SIDE THEN ON THE OTHER.

BODY PART WORKED
Outer Thigh (Abductor)

SET UP
Lie on your side, with the top arm supporting the weight in front of your body. Hips and legs should be directly on top of each other and knees should be bent at a 90-degree angle. Hold abdominal muscles in tight.

TIPS FROM JONI
Be sure to keep your hips stacked directly on top of each other for maximum effectiveness.

Circuit Two

35

BODY PART WORKED

Lower Back (Erector Spinae)

SET UP

Lie face down with your legs extended straight and arms extended overhead.

TIPS FROM JONI

This is a great move to strengthen the lower back. Perform this move very smoothly, flowing into the position.

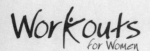

Superwoman

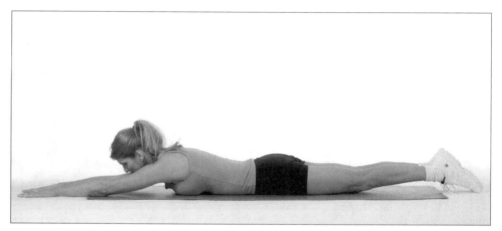

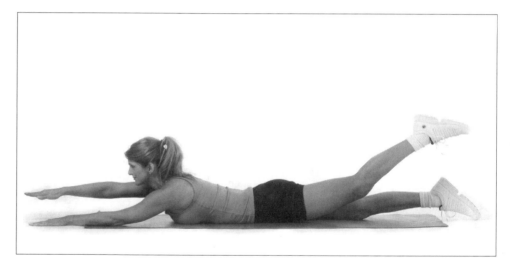

Exercise Technique

1. Exhale as you lift the opposite arm and opposite leg simultaneously, holding for a moment.

2. Slowly lower back to start and smoothly follow with the same motion, using the opposite arm and leg.

REPEAT A TOTAL OF 16 TIMES ALTERNATING RIGHT AND LEFT.

Pulse-up Crunches

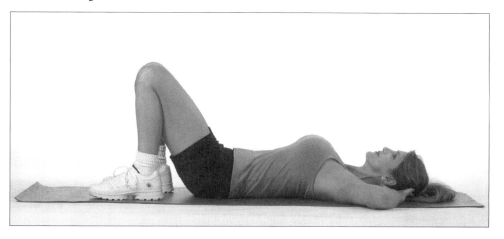

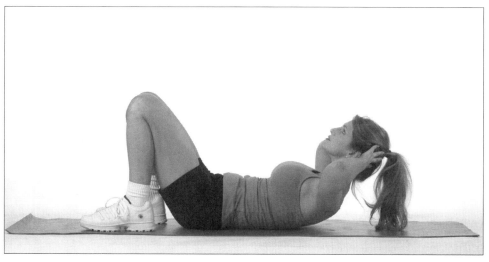

Exercise Technique

1. Exhale and lift your shoulder blades up and forward while contracting your abdomen in a pulsing up-and-down motion without allowing your head to rest back down in between pulses.

REPEAT 20 TO 30 TIMES.

SET UP
Lie flat on your back with your knees bent, heels close to your body, and pelvis tilted slightly upward to help flatten the back. Place your fingertips lightly against the back of your head.

TIPS FROM JONI
Keep your elbows back and out of sight. Focus your eyes upward and keep your chin one fist distance off your chest at all times.

Circuit Two

THREE

EQUIPMENT
Dumbbells
Ankle Weights
Chair

CIRCUIT

Workouts for Women

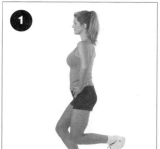

Samba   **PG 39**

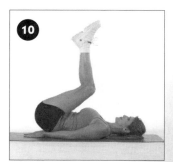

Marches   **PG 40**

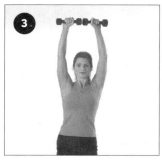

Rotating Overhead Press **PG 41**

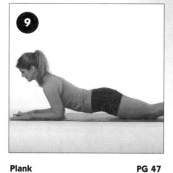

Reverse Curl   **PG 48**

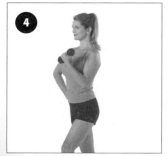

Single Biceps Curl   **PG 42**

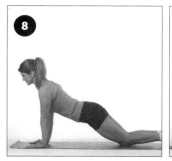

Plank   **PG 47**

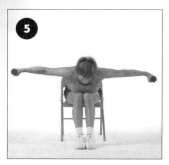

Seated Bent-over Arc   **PG 43**

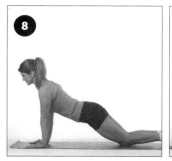

Triceps Push-Ups   **PG 46**

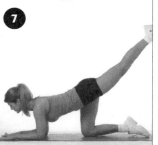

Kneeling Straight-Leg Glute **PG 45**

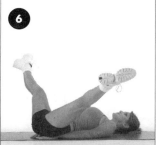

Lying Inner Thigh V   **PG 44**

Samba

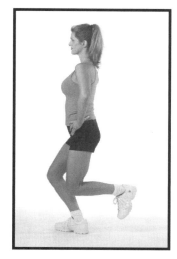 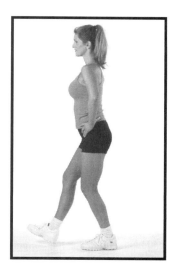

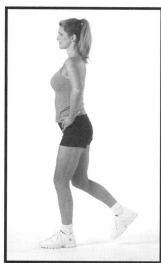 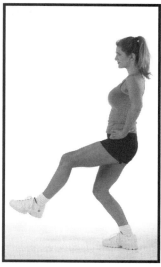

BODY PART WORKED
Cardiovascular System

SET UP
Stand tall with shoulders back, chest high, and abdomen in tight.

TIPS FROM JONI
Let your arms move with you and enjoy this fun cardiovascular move.

Exercise Technique

1. Step forward on one leg, swaying your hip into the direction of your step, tap the opposite leg in place then step back with the forward leg swaying your hip into the opposite direction.

COMPLETE SEVERAL FORWARD AND BACK SETS ON ONE SIDE, THEN SWITCH TO THE OTHER SIDE ALTERNATING FOR ABOUT 2 MINUTES.

Circuit Three

SET UP
Stand tall, holding a chair
for balance, with knees
slightly bent and ankle
weights around ankles.
Pull shoulders back, hold
chest high, and hold
abdominal muscles in
tight.

TIPS FROM JONI
Keep toes pointed
throughout the move.
Hold abdominal muscles in
tight and keep shoulders
back.

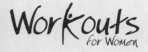

Marches

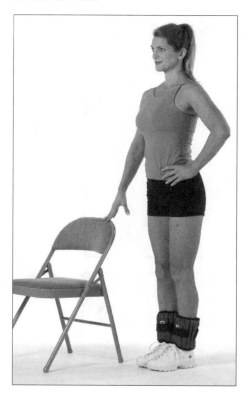
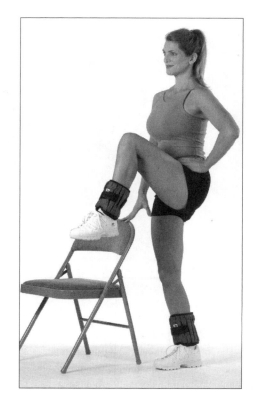

Exercise Technique
1. Exhale as you lift one knee up toward your chest.

2. Lower your leg, tapping your toes onto the floor momentarily, then repeat.

REPEAT 15 TIMES ON ONE SIDE THEN 15 ON THE OTHER.

Rotating Overhead Press

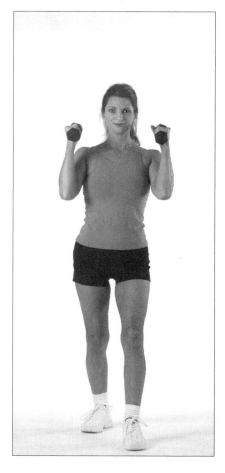 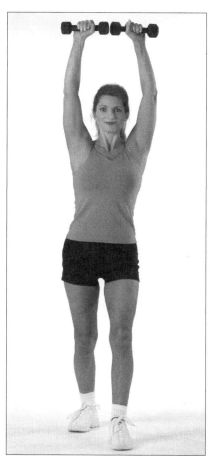

SET UP
Stand tall with abdominal muscles held in tight and dumbbells in both hands. Bend arms at the elbows and pull elbows in close to your body with hands at about shoulder height with palms facing in toward you.

TIPS FROM JONI
When extending arms overhead be sure not to overextend by keeping elbows soft.

Exercise Technique

1. Exhale as you extend your arms straight up overhead, rotating the palms so that they are facing forward at the top.

2. Lower your arms down to start while simultaneously rotating palms back in.

REPEAT 15 TIMES.

Circuit Three

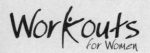

Single Biceps Curl

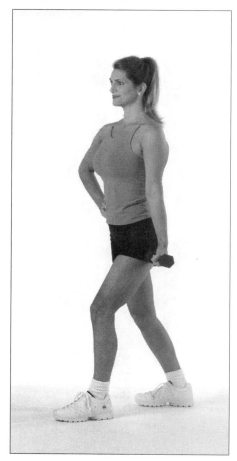 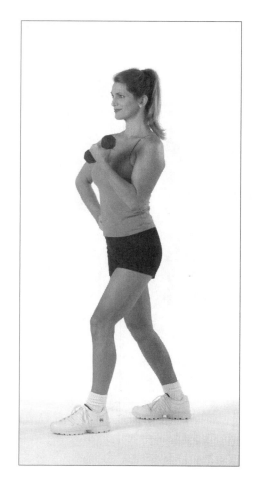

Exercise Technique

1. Exhale as you bend your arm at the elbow, bringing the hand up toward your shoulder with the palm facing your chest at the top of the move.

2. Extend your arm back down to start in a controlled manner.

REPEAT 15 TIMES ON ONE SIDE THEN ON THE OTHER.

Seated Bent-over Arc

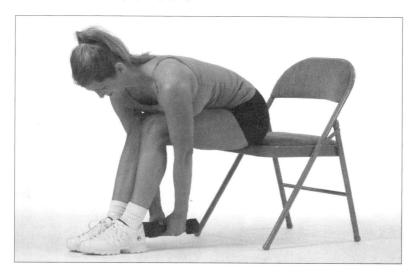

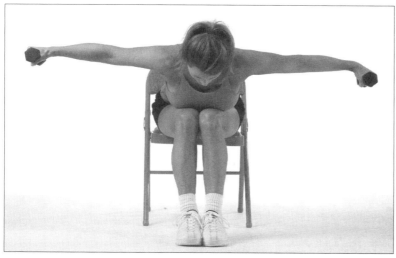

Exercise Technique

1. Exhale as you bring your arms straight out to the sides in an arc, squeezing your shoulder blades together at the top of the move.

2. Reverse the move and lower your arms back to start in a controlled manner.

REPEAT 15 TIMES.

BODY PART WORKED
Back and Rear Shoulders, Back (Posterior Deltoid, Trapezius)

SET UP
Hold a dumbbell in each hand and sit on the edge of a chair. Bend forward at the hips. Rest your chest on your thighs with your arms hanging at your side, palms facing in toward each other. Hold abdominal muscles in tight.

TIPS FROM JONI
Be sure not to use momentum during this move. Focus on using your back muscles during the lifting phase.

Circuit Three

SET UP

Lie on your back with your hands under your hips, which will tilt your pelvis slightly upward and flatten your back. Bring your legs together and straight up with feet flexed.

TIPS FROM JONI

Lead with your heels as you bring your legs back in to start to keep the move focused and effective for the inner thigh.

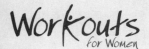

Lying Inner Thigh V

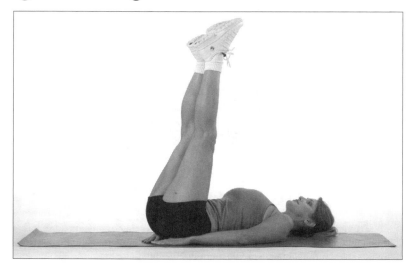

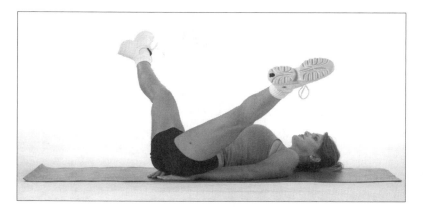

Exercise Technique

1. In a very controlled manner, let your legs come apart as far as you can comfortably go.

2. Exhale as you bring your legs back in together.

REPEAT 15 TIMES.

Kneeling Straight-Leg Glute

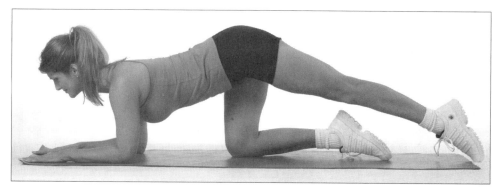

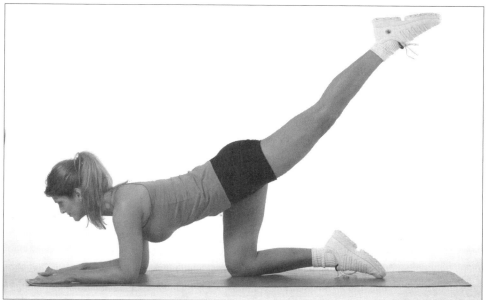

SET UP
Kneel down on your elbows and knees. Extend one leg back with toes pointed. Hold your abdomen in tight.

TIPS FROM JONI
Keep hips square to the floor throughout the move.

Exercise Technique

1. Exhale as you lift the extended leg up as high as possible, squeezing the buttocks at the top of the move.

2. Bring the extended leg back down, momentarily tapping your toes lightly on the floor.

REPEAT 15 TIMES ON ONE SIDE THEN ON THE OTHER.

Circuit Three

BODY PART WORKED

Chest, Back of Arms
(Pectoral, Triceps)

SET UP

Kneel down on the floor on your hands and knees, with your hands directly under your shoulders and fingers facing forward. Hold your abdomen in tight.

TIPS FROM JONI

Be careful not to lock your elbows as you push back up to start. Keep your neck in line with your spine throughout the move.

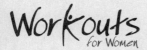

Triceps Push-Ups

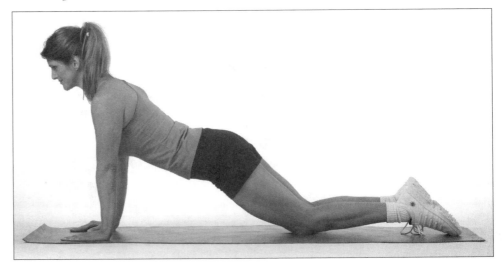

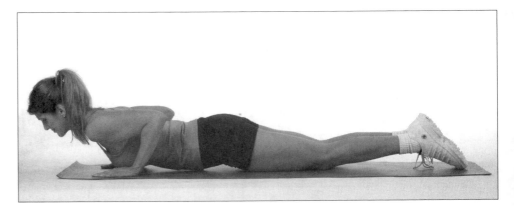

Exercise Technique

1. Bend at the elbows and lower your chest, stopping one fist distance from the floor.

2. Exhale as you push back up to start by straightening your arms.

REPEAT 15 TIMES.

Plank

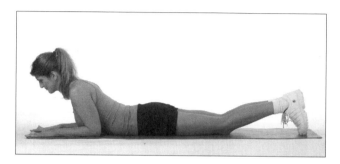

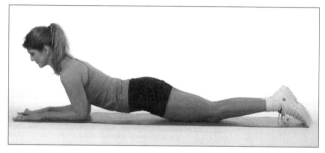

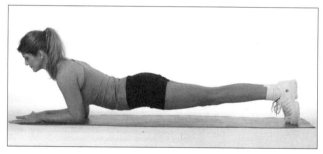

BODY PART WORKED
Core Muscles, Including Trunk and Pelvis (Rectus Abdominis and Transverse Abdominis)

SET UP
Lie face down on the floor with your elbows bent right next to your chest resting on your forearms with palms facing down.

TIPS FROM JONI
During the exercise a common tendency is to hold your breath. Be sure to breathe normally throughout the move.

Exercise Technique

1. Lift your midsection up off the floor and rise up onto your knees first, then up to your toes and forearms, keeping your back and buttocks flat from knees to shoulders.

2. Hold this position for 15 seconds, keeping your abdomen held in tight.

3. Slowly and carefully come back down onto your knees, and move right back into set-up position, resting for 5 seconds before lifting up again.

REPEAT 3 TIMES.

Circuit Three

BODY PART WORKED

Lower Abdomen (Rectus Abdominis)

SET UP

Lie on your back with your hands under the buttocks to lift the pelvis up slightly and flatten the back. Place your feet flat on the floor with your knees bent.

TIPS FROM JONI

Be sure not to rock your body to lift your legs up. Use your abdominal muscles to lift your pelvis and buttocks which will keep the focus on the lower abdominal muscles.

Workouts *for Women*

Reverse Curl

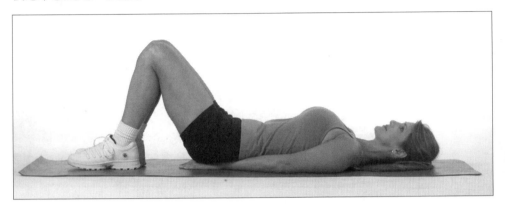

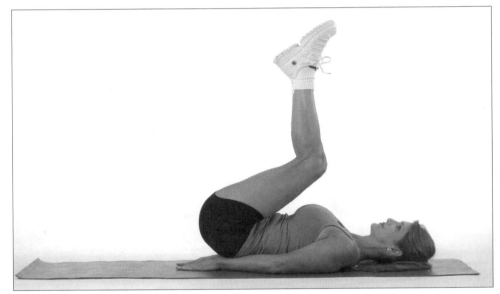

Exercise Technique

1. Keeping knees bent and together, exhale as you lift the pelvis and buttocks up off the floor, bringing knees in toward the chest.

2. Still keeping knees bent and together, reverse the move by rolling the pelvis and buttocks back toward the floor. As your feet come back toward the floor, momentarily tap your toes onto the floor then, repeat the move.

REPEAT 15 TIMES.

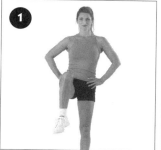

**Alternating Knee Up,
Then Squat**   **PG 50**

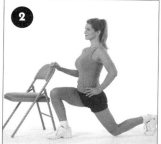

Alternating Reverse Lunge   **PG 51**

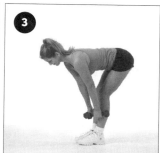

Dead Lift   **PG 52**

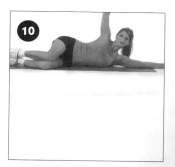

Oblique Reach   **PG 59**

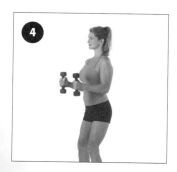

Halfway Up Hammer Curl   **PG 53**

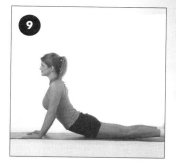

Belly-Ups   **PG 58**

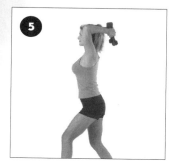

Overhead Triceps Extension   **PG 54**

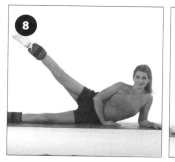

Lying Straight-Leg Outer Thigh   **PG 57**

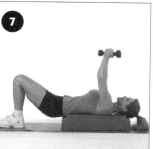

Chest Flies on Step   **PG 56**

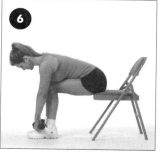

Seated Forward Raise   **PG 55**

EQUIPMENT
Step
Dumbbells
Ankle Weights
Chair

Circuit Four

SET UP

Stand tall with shoulders back, chest high, and abdomen held in tight, with hands on your waist. Legs should be outside shoulder width apart.

TIPS FROM JONI

Be sure that as you squat down your knees do not extend over your toes or you will be placing too much stress on your knees.

Alternating Knee Up, Then Squat

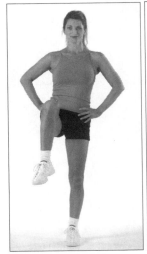
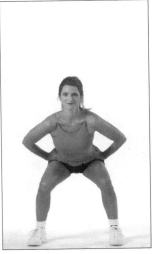
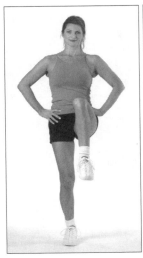
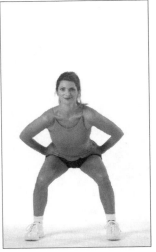

Exercise Technique

1. Bring one knee up to your chest.

2. Lower the leg down as you sit back into a squat by bending both knees and reaching back with your buttocks as if you were sitting on a chair behind you.

3. Bring the opposite leg up to your chest then, lower down into squat position on the other side.

REPEAT FOR TWO MINUTES.

Workouts for Women

Alternating Reverse Lunge

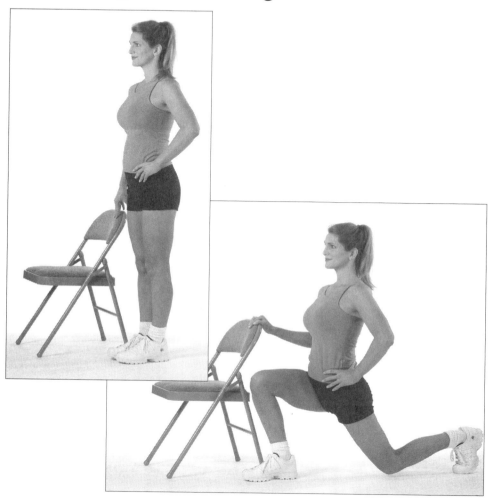

SET UP
Stand up straight and tall with legs together, shoulders back, chest high, and abdomen held in tight. Position a chair next to you to hold onto for balance.

TIPS FROM JONI
As you lower down, the front knee should always be directly over your ankle and not over your toes or you will be placing too much pressure on the knee.

Exercise Technique

1. Take a slow, controlled step back with one leg, landing on the ball of the foot.

2. Bend both knees while lowering your hips toward the floor, stopping before the back knee touches the floor.

3. Exhale as you push off the trailing foot and the front heel as you straighten your legs to return to starting position.

REPEAT 15 TIMES ON ONE SIDE THEN ON THE OTHER SIDE.

Circuit Four

BODY PART WORKED

Back of Legs, Lower Back (Hamstring, Erector Spinae)

SET UP

Stand tall with shoulders back, chest high, and abdominal muscles held in tight. Position feet loosely together with dumbbells in hands and arms hanging straight at your sides, with palms facing in toward your body.

TIPS FROM JONI

Keep your hands very close to your body throughout the entire move as if you were shaving your legs.

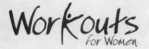

Dead Lift

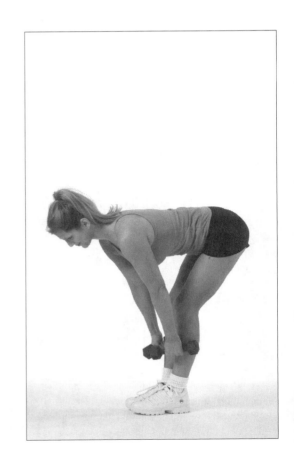

Exercise Technique

1. Keep a slight bend in your knees as you bend forward at the hip, reaching back with your tailbone, allowing your hands to move downward toward your feet.

2. Stop at the point at which you feel slight tension in the back of your legs, then exhale as you stand back up returning to start.

REPEAT 15 TIMES.

Halfway Up Hammer Curl

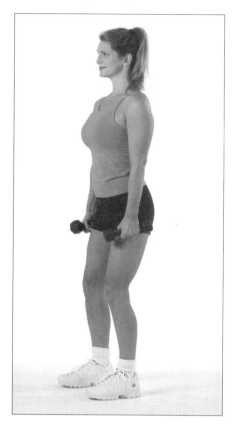 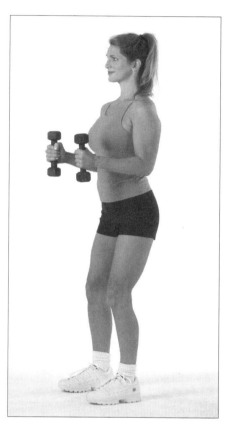

BODY PART WORKED

Front of Arms (Biceps)

SET UP

Stand with dumbbells in hands with feet shoulder width apart. Place your arms down at your sides with the palms facing in. Hold your shoulders back, chest high, and your abdominal muscles in tight.

TIPS FROM JONI

Keep elbows stationary at your sides throughout the move, being sure they do not move forward or backward.

Exercise Technique

1. Keep your elbows stationary and at your sides as you bend your arms at the elbows, lifting arms halfway up until forearms are parallel to the floor.

2. Extend arms back down to your sides in a controlled manner.

REPEAT 15 TIMES.

Circuit Four

SET UP

Stand tall with abdominal muscles held in tight, shoulders back and chest high, holding dumbbells in each hand. Lift your arms directly overhead with elbows close to your ears.

TIPS FROM JONI

Be sure your elbows do not drift, keeping them close to your ears and stationary.

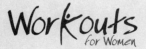

Overhead Triceps Extension

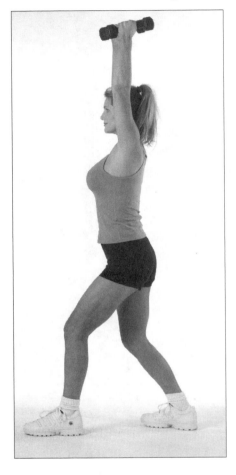 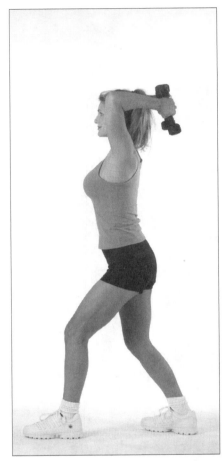

Exercise Technique

1. Bend at the elbows as you lower the weight toward the back of your neck.

2. Exhale as you press arms straight up to start position, feeling the tension in the back of the arms.

REPEAT 15 TIMES.

Seated Forward Raise

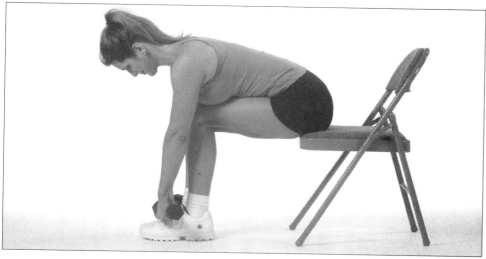

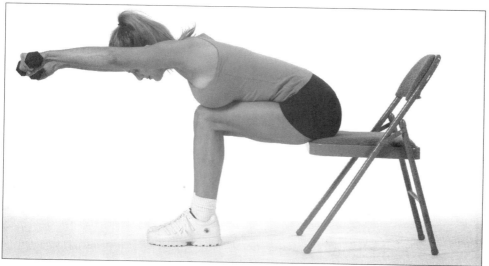

SET UP
Sit on the edge of a chair. Bend forward at the hips and rest your chest on your thighs, with your arms hanging toward the floor in front of your legs, holding dumbbells in both hands with palms facing in toward each other. Hold abdominal muscles in tight.

TIPS FROM JONI
Use very light weights for this exercise, being careful not to strain the neck or upper back.

Exercise Technique
1. Exhale as you lift arms straight out in front up to shoulder level.

2. Lower back down to start in a controlled manner.

REPEAT 15 TIMES.

Circuit Four

SET UP

Lie on top of the step with your neck and back supported. Start with your arms straight up, directly over your chest, with dumbbell in each hand and palms facing in toward each other.

TIPS FROM JONI

Be sure not to let your back arch and lift off the step as you lower the weight downward.

Workouts for Women

56

Chest Flies on Step

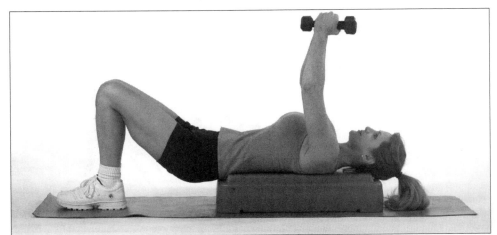

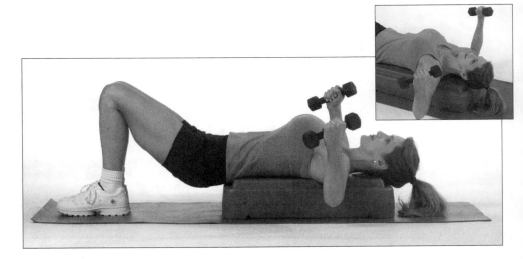

Exercise Technique

1. Bend arms at the elbows out in an arc as you lower the weight down, stopping when you feel a slight stretch through the chest.

2. Exhale and reverse the arc as you lift the weight back up to start position in a controlled manner.

REPEAT 15 TIMES.

Lying Straight-Leg Outer Thigh

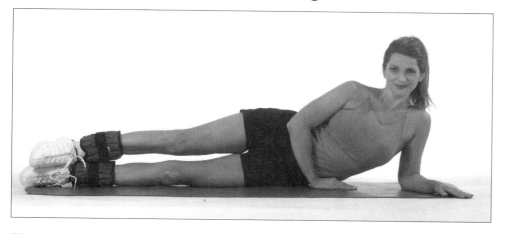

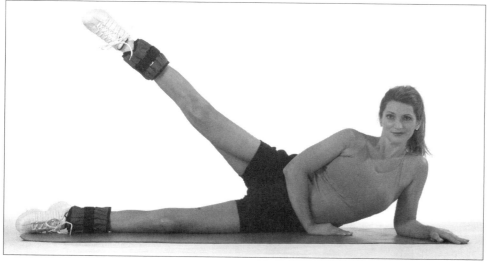

Exercise Technique

1. Exhale and lead with the heel as you lift the top leg as high as you comfortably can.

2. Lower the leg back down in a controlled manner without resting it on the other leg.

REPEAT 15 TIMES ON ONE SIDE THEN ON THE OTHER.

Circuit Four

Workouts for Women

58

Belly-Ups

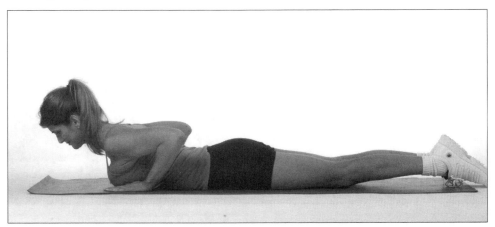

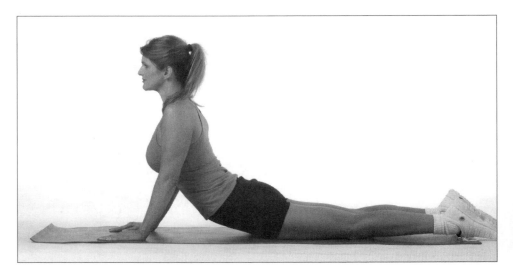

Exercise Technique

1. Exhale as you straighten your arms, lifting your chest off the floor and arching your back, stopping before you feel any discomfort in your back.

2. Bend elbows as you lower back down to starting position in a controlled manner.

REPEAT 10 TO 15 TIMES.

Oblique Reach

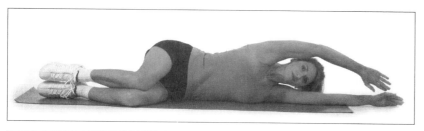

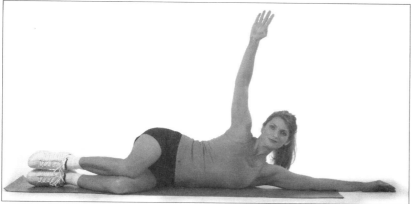

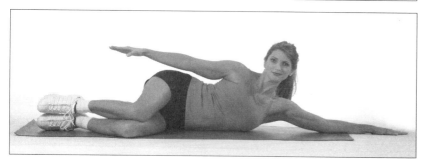

SET UP
Lie on your side with knees bent and stacked directly on top of each other. Extend both arms overhead.

TIPS FROM JONI
Perform this move in a pulsing motion.

Exercise Technique

1. Exhale as you reach forward with the top arm, lifting shoulder up and forward towards your hips.

2. Lower shoulder back toward the floor without resting your head or shoulder down on the floor.

REPEAT 10 TO 15 TIMES ON ONE SIDE BEFORE SWITCHING TO THE OTHER.

FIVE

EQUIPMENT

Step
Dumbbells
Ankle Weights

Workouts for Women

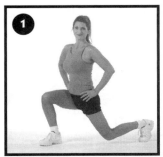

Cardio Lunges PG 61

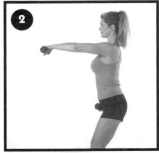

Alternating Forward Raises PG 62

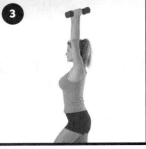

Overhead Triceps Extension PG 63

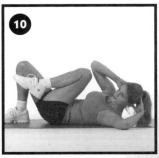

Oblique Pulses PG 70

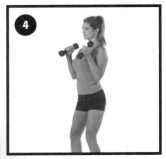

Hammer Curls PG 64

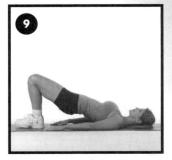

Pelvic Tilt PG 69

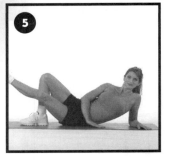

Inner Thigh Lift PG 65

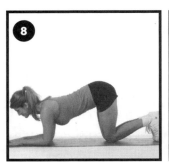

Prone Leg Press PG 68

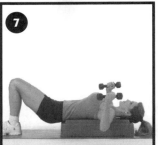

Chest Press on Step PG 67

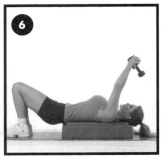

Straight-Arm Pullover on Step PG 66

Cardio Lunges

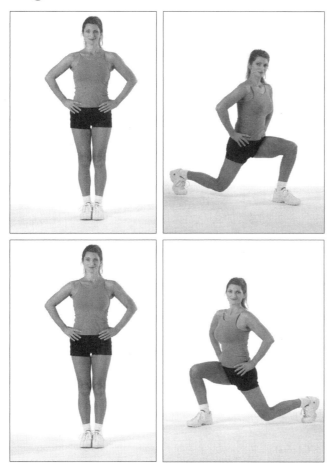

SET UP
Stand tall with legs together, shoulders back, chest out high, and abdominal muscles held in tight. Place hands on your waist.

TIPS FROM JONI
Be sure that as you step out to the side that you do not allow your knee to extend past the toes, or you will be putting too much pressure on the knees.

Exercise Technique

1. Take a long step out to the side with one leg, turning the foot outward and shifting your body weight in the same direction as you bend the knee. Keep the stationary leg straight.

2. Exhale as you press up with the heel and pull the leg back in to start.

3. Take a very slight hop as you proceed to repeat the long step out to the side with the opposite leg.

PERFORM THIS EXERCISE AT A MODERATE PACE, WITH A SLIGHT HOP BETWEEN EACH MOVE MAKING THIS AN AEROBIC-PACED MOVEMENT, FOR TWO MINUTES.

Circuit Five

Front of Shoulders
(Posterior Deltoid)

SET UP

Stand tall with abdominal muscles held in tight, shoulders back, and chest high. Hold a dumbbell in each hand with your palms resting on your thighs in front of your body.

TIPS FROM JONI

Keep a slight bend in your knees during this move to release some pressure from your back, as you lift the weight up in front of your body.

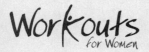

Alternating Forward Raises

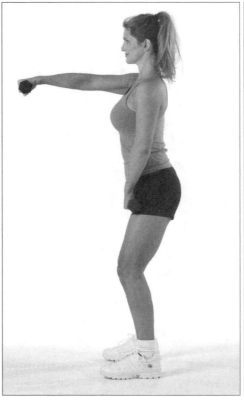 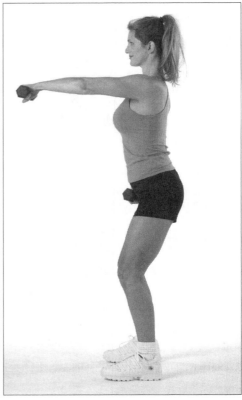

Exercise Technique

1. Exhale as you raise one arm directly in front of your body, stopping at shoulder height.

2. Lower arm back down in a controlled manner and repeat on the other side.

REPEAT A TOTAL OF 30 TIMES ALTERNATING RIGHT AND LEFT.

Overhead Triceps Extension

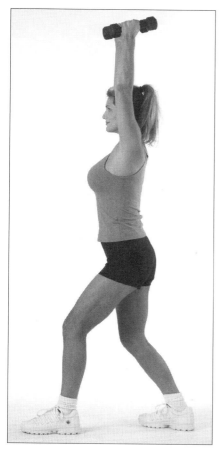 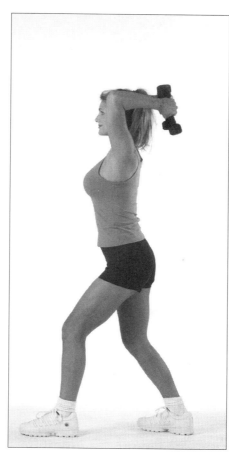

SET UP
Stand tall with abdominal muscles held in tight, shoulders back, and chest high. Hold dumbbells in each hand. Lift your arms directly overhead with elbows close to your ears.

TIPS FROM JONI
Be sure elbows do not drift, keeping them close to your ears and stationary.

Exercise Technique
1. Bend at the elbows as you lower the weight toward the back of your neck.

2. Exhale as you press arms straight up to start position, feeling the tension in the back of the arms.

REPEAT 15 TIMES.

Circuit Five

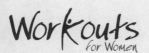
Hammer Curls

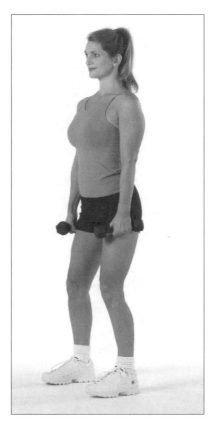
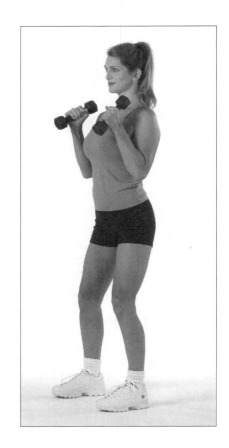

Exercise Technique

1. Exhale as you bend your arms at the elbows, lifting hands up toward your shoulders.

2. Extend arms back down to your sides in a controlled manner.

REPEAT 15 TIMES.

Inner Thigh Lift

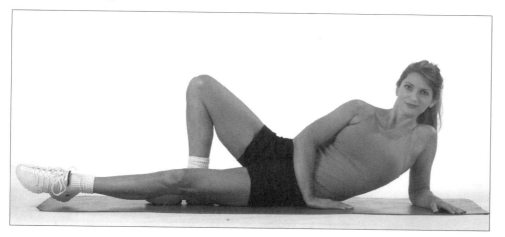

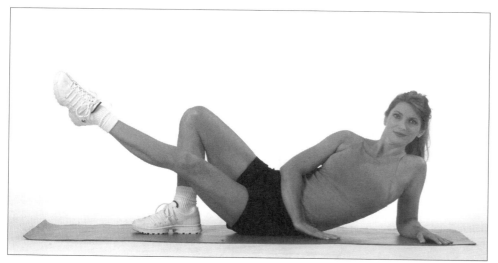

SET UP
Lie on your side with your bottom leg extended and the top leg bent, with foot flat on the floor behind the bottom leg. Shift your body weight onto the lower hip and prop your body up with the corresponding forearm.

TIPS FROM JONI
It's important to keep the heel of the extended leg rotated upward to keep the focus on the inner thigh.

Exercise Technique
1. With the foot flexed and heel rotated upward, exhale and lift the extended leg upward as high as you can comfortably go.
2. Lower the leg back down in a controlled manner without touching the floor.

REPEAT 15 TIMES ON ONE SIDE THEN ON THE OTHER.

Circuit Five

SET UP

Lie on the step with your back and neck supported, with both arms extended upward with both hands holding onto one dumbbell.

TIPS FROM JONI

Be sure not to let your back arch and come off of the step as you lower the weight behind you.

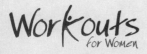

Straight-Arm Pullover on Step

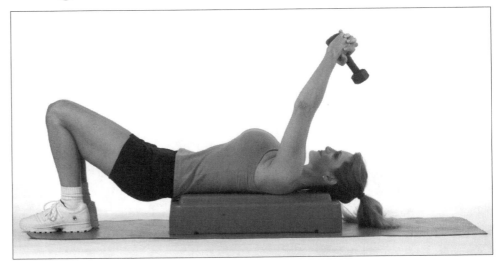

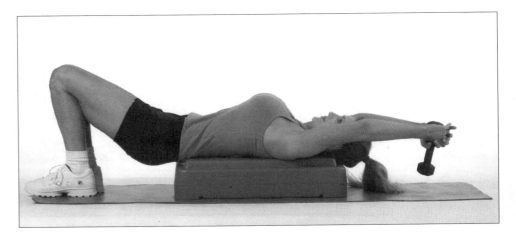

Exercise Technique

1. Keeping your arms almost straight and your back flat, lower the weight back and down overhead in an arc until you feel a slight stretch through your arms and chest.

2. Exhale and pull the weight back up to start in a controlled manner.

REPEAT 15 TIMES.

Chest Press on Step

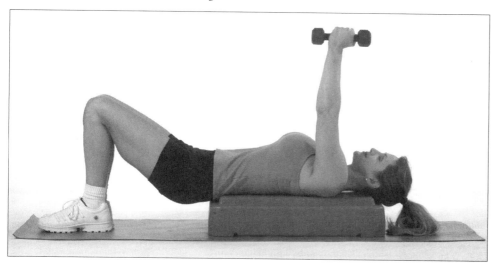

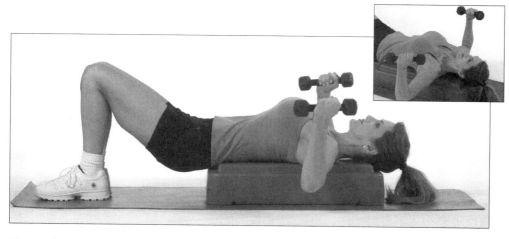

Exercise Technique

1. Bend at the elbows as you lower the weight straight downward, stopping when you feel a stretch through the chest.

2. Exhale as you extend your arms, pressing the weight straight back up to start.

REPEAT 15 TIMES.

BODY PART WORKED
Chest (Pectoral)

SET UP
Lie on a step with your back flat and neck supported. Hold a dumbbell in each hand and extend both arms straight up from your shoulders in line with your chest, with palms facing in toward each other.

TIPS FROM JONI
Keep your wrists straight throughout the move.

Circuit Five

67

SET UP

Kneel down on your hands
and knees with abdomen
held in tight. Your knees
should be together and
directly under your hips,
and your fingers should be
pointing straight ahead.

TIPS FROM JONI

Be sure to maintain proper
breathing during this
move since the tendency
can be to hold your
breath.

Workouts for Women

Prone Leg Press

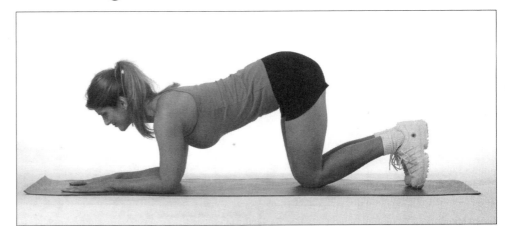

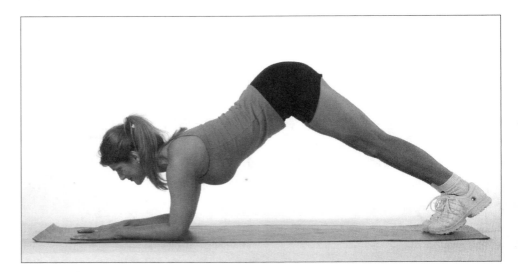

Exercise Technique

1. Exhale as you straighten your knees and tighten the front of your thighs at
   the top of the move.

2. Reverse the move and bend at the knees, stopping just before your knees
   touch the floor.

REPEAT 15 TIMES.

Pelvic Tilt

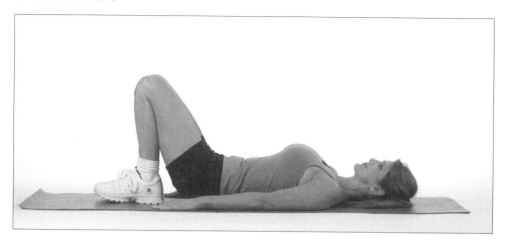

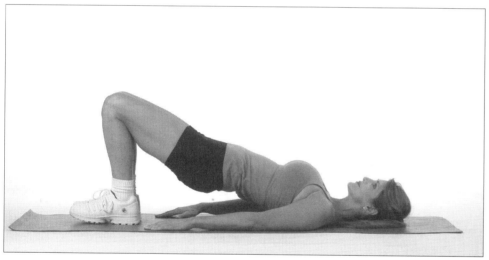

Exercise Technique

1. Exhale as you raise your hips, keeping the upper back on the ground. Tighten the buttocks as you rise.

2. Lower your hips back down in a controlled manner, momentarily touching hips to the floor before repeating.

REPEAT 15 TIMES.

SET UP
Lie on your back with your knees bent and heels pressing into the floor.

TIPS FROM JONI
Contracting your buttocks at the top of the move as your raise your hips upward will maximize the effectiveness of this move.

Circuit Five

SET UP

Lie on your back with knees bent and heels close to your body. Tilt the pelvis up slightly to flatten out your back. Place fingertips lightly against the back of your head.

TIPS FROM JONI

Be sure not to allow the faster pace of this move to compromise your form.

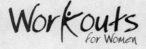

Oblique Pulses

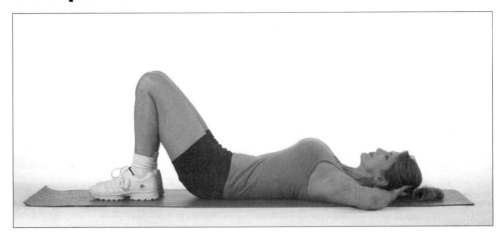

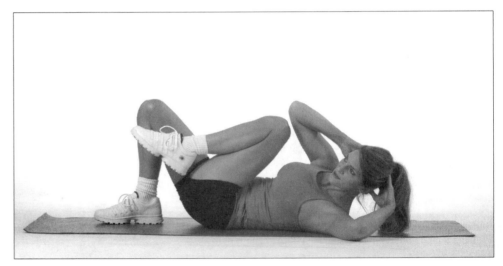

Exercise Technique

1. Exhale as you lift and rotate one shoulder toward the opposite knee.

2. Lower shoulder back down to start position, then immediately perform the move on the opposite side.

PERFORM THIS MOVE IN A FAST PACED PULSING MOTION, ALTERNATING FROM SIDE TO SIDE FOR A TOTAL OF 20 TO 30 TIMES.

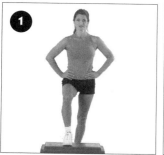
Alternating Step Up PG 72

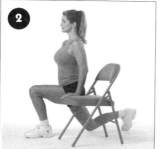
Alternating Forward Lunge PG 73

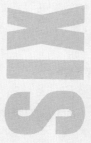
Bent-over Arc PG 74

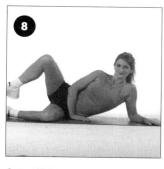
Reverse Bicycle Crunch PG 81

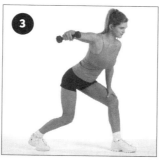
Rotating Biceps Curl PG 75

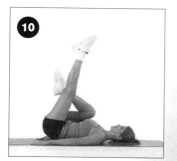
Elevated Pelvic Tilt PG 80

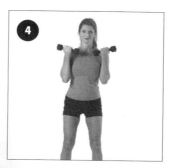
Rotating Overhead Press PG 76

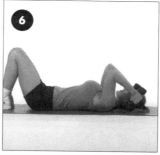
Outer Thigh Rotator PG 79

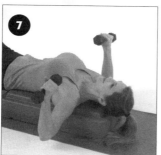
Palm-out Chest Press on Step PG 78

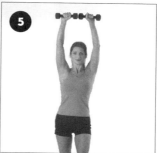
Lying Triceps Extension PG 77

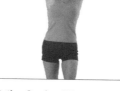

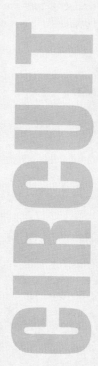

EQUIPMENT
Step
Dumbbells
Ankle Weights
Chair

Circuit Six

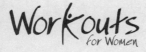

Alternating Step Up

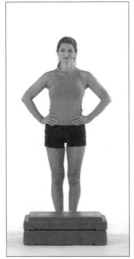
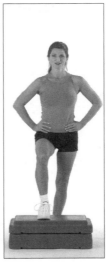
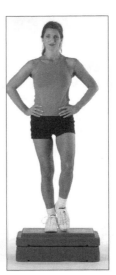
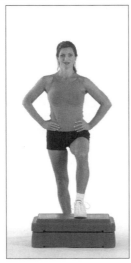
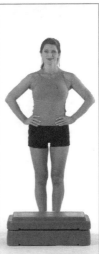

Exercise Technique

1. Step right foot up onto the step, landing first with the heel.

2. Tap up onto step with the toes of the left foot.

3. Step down onto the floor with the left foot, then the right foot so that you are back where you started with both feet on the floor.

REPEAT, ALTERNATING THE RIGHT AND LEFT SIDE AT A MODERATE PACE FOR ABOUT 2 MINUTES TO INCREASE YOUR HEART RATE.

Alternating Forward Lunge

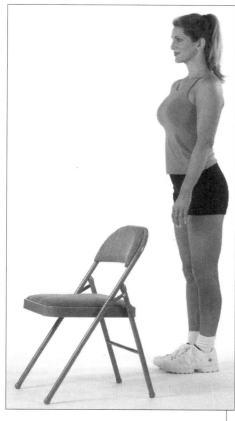

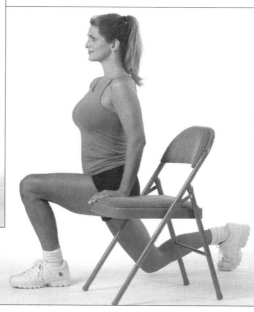

SET UP
Start standing tall with
feet together and abdomi-
nal muscles held in tight,
shoulders back and chest
out. Hold onto a chair for
balance if you need to.

TIPS FROM JONI
As you lower down, be
sure the front knee does
not extend past your toes
or you will be putting too
much pressure on your
knees.

Exercise Technique

1. Take a long step forward with one leg, landing first with the heel.

2. As the forward foot hits the floor, immediately bend at the knees, lowering hips toward the floor.

3. Push off the front heel and return to start.

REPEAT A TOTAL OF 20 TIMES ALTERNATING RIGHT AND LEFT.

Circuit Six

SET UP

Begin this exercise in a semi-lunge position, standing with one leg forward and one back. Both knees should be pointing straight ahead and abdominal muscles should be held in tight. Lean forward, bending at the hip, and rest the forward hand on your forward thigh to support your body. Hold a dumbbell in the other hand and position the arm hanging down holding the weight near the forward knee.

TIPS FROM JONI

Be sure to keep your forward hand on the thigh to support your back throughout the move.

Workouts for Women

Bent-over Arc

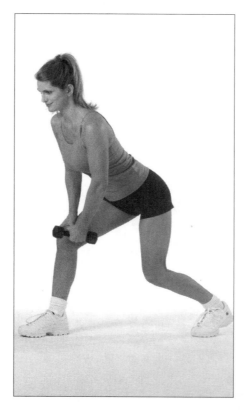 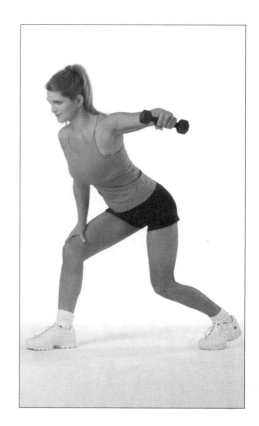

Exercise Technique

1. Exhale as you lift the weight out to the side in a wide arc, stopping at about shoulder height, squeezing the shoulder blades together at the top of the movement.

2. Reverse the arc, lowering the weight back down toward the forward knee, returning to start.

REPEAT 15 TIMES ON ONE SIDE THEN ON THE OTHER.

Rotating Biceps Curl

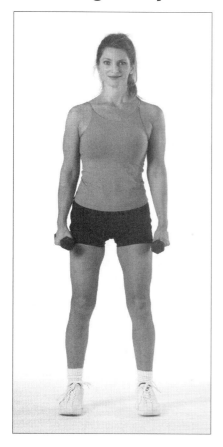 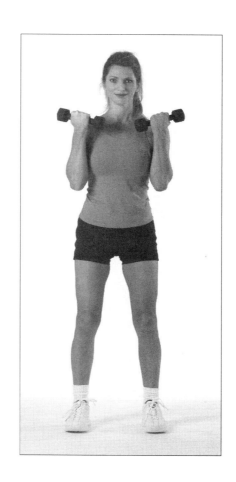

BODY PART WORKED
Front of Arms (Biceps)

SET UP
Stand tall with shoulders back, chest high and abdominal muscles held in tight. Hold a dumbbell in each hand with arms down at your sides with palms facing in towards you.

TIPS FROM JONI
Keep elbows stationary at your sides throughout the move.

Exercise Technique

1. Exhale and bend arms at the elbows and lift both hands up toward your shoulders, rotating the hands so that palms are facing toward your shoulders at the top of the move.

2. Reverse the motion, lowering your hands back down, rotating hands so that palms are facing in again at the bottom of the move.

REPEAT 15 TIMES.

SET UP

Start standing tall with dumbbells in both hands with arms bent at the elbows and hands at shoulder level with palms facing in. Hold abdominal muscles in tight, shoulders back, and chest high.

TIPS FROM JONI

Be sure not to overextend the elbows at the top of the move.

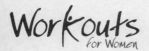

Rotating Overhead Press

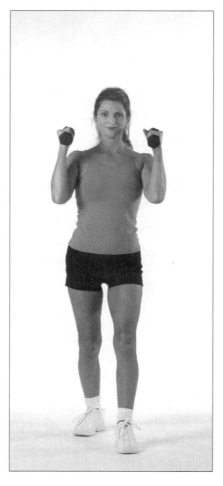 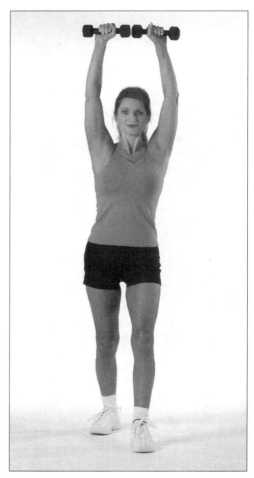

Exercise Technique

1. Exhale as you extend your arms straight overhead, rotating palms so that they are facing forward at the top.

2. Reverse the motion, lowering your hands back down and rotating hands so that palms are facing in again at the bottom of the move.

REPEAT 15 TIMES.

Lying Triceps Extension

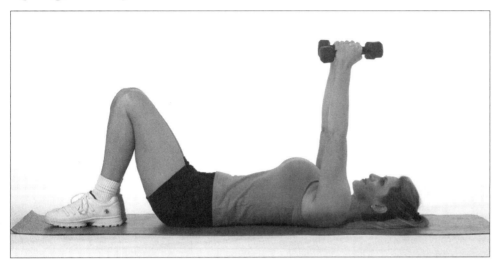

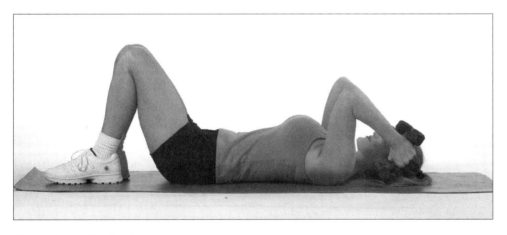

Exercise Technique

1. Keep upper arms motionless as you bend at the elbows, lowering the weight toward your shoulders, feeling the tension in the back of your arms.

2. Still keeping upper arms motionless, exhale and extend arms back up to start.

REPEAT 15 TIMES.

SET UP
Lie flat on your back with knees bent and feet flat on the floor. With dumbbells in both hands, extend your arms straight up from the shoulders.

TIPS FROM JONI
Keeping upper arms motionless on both the lifting and lowering phase is critical to making this exercise effective. If your arms drift forward or back the focus will not remain on the back of the arms as intended.

Circuit Six

BODY PART WORKED
Chest (Pectoral)

SET UP
Lie on a step with your back flat and neck supported. Hold a dumbbell in each hand and extend both arms straight up from your shoulders in line with your chest, with palms facing away from you.

TIPS FROM JONI
Be sure not to overextend the elbows at the top of the move.

Workouts for Women

78

Palm-out Chest Press on Step

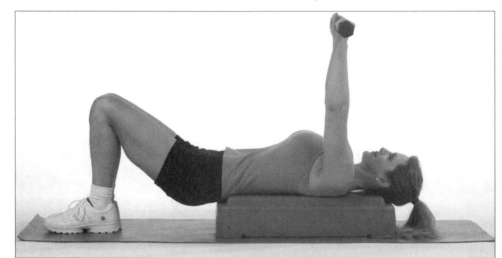

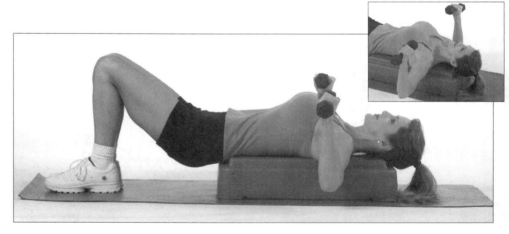

Exercise Technique
1. Bend at the elbows as you lower the weight straight downward, stopping when you feel a stretch through the chest.

2. Exhale as you extend your arms, pressing the weight straight back up to start.

REPEAT 15 TIMES.

Outer Thigh Rotator

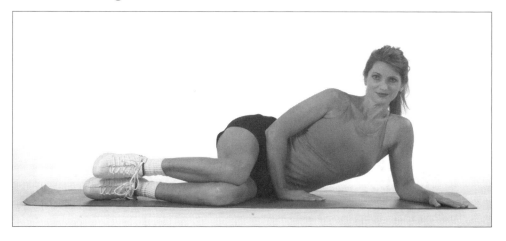

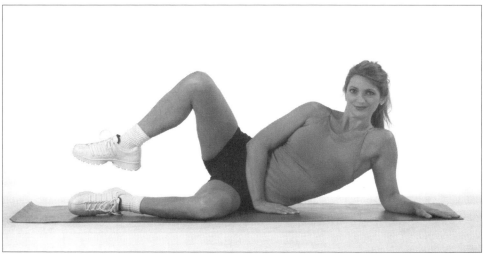

BODY PART WORKED
Outer Thigh (Abductor)

SET UP
Lie on your side, with the top arm supporting you in front of your body. Hips and legs should be directly on top of each other and knees should be bent at a 90-degree angle.

TIPS FROM JONI
Be sure to keep your hips stacked directly on top of each other for maximum effectiveness.

Exercise Technique

1. Keeping feet close together, exhale as you lift the top leg in an arc as high as you can comfortably go.

2. Still keeping feet close together, control the leg as you lower back to start without resting the leg down.

REPEAT 15 TIMES ON ONE SIDE THEN ON THE OTHER.

Circuit Six

SET UP
Place a step in front of you with the long side facing you. Lie on your back right behind the step with knees bent, and heels pressing into the step. Feet should be close together with knees apart.

TIPS FROM JONI
For maximum effectiveness, you must contract the buttocks on the lifting motion.

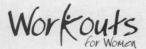

Elevated Pelvic Tilt

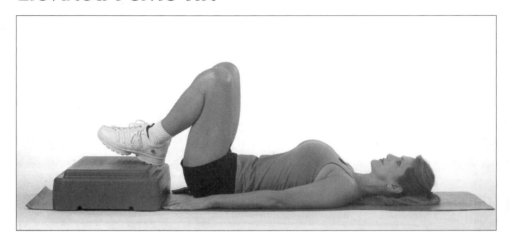

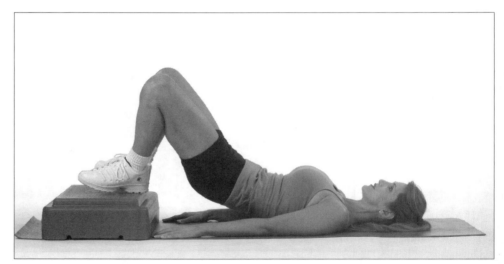

Exercise Technique
1. Dig heels into step and exhale as you raise hips off the floor, keeping upper back on the ground, tightening buttocks as you rise.

2. Lower hips back down in a controlled manner, momentarily touching hips to the floor before repeating.

REPEAT 15 TIMES.

Reverse Bicycle Crunch

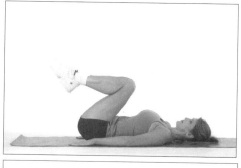 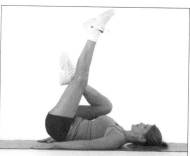

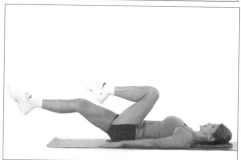 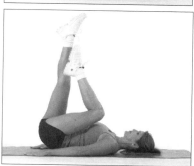

Exercise Technique

1. Exhale as you extend one leg straight up as you simultaneously lift the pelvis up.

2. Lower the leg and the pelvis down, bringing the knee in toward the chest, and when you are midway back to start position, begin to extend the other leg straight up as you simultaneously lift up the pelvis.

ALTERNATE RIGHT AND LEFT FOR A TOTAL OF 20 TO 30 TIMES.

BODY PART WORKED
Lower Abdomen (Rectus Abdominis)

SET UP
Lie flat on your back with both legs lifted up with knees bent and together. Place your hands at your sides with palms facing down.

TIPS FROM JONI
Lifting up with the pelvis is what creates the focus on your abdominal muscles. Be sure not to initiate the lift by using rocking and momentum.

Circuit Six

SEVEN

EQUIPMENT
Dumbbells
Ankle Weights
Chair

Workouts *for Women*

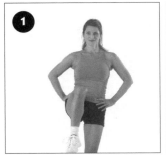
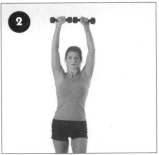

Knee Up / Curl Back Combo   PG 83

Rotate-in Overhead Press   PG 85

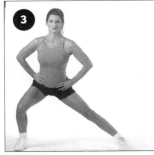

Side Lunge   PG 86

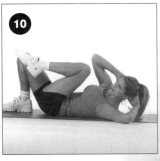

Knee-in Oblique   PG 93

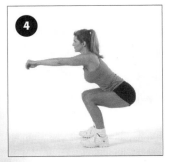

Squats   PG 87

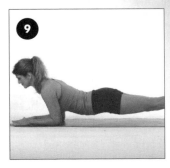

Plank   PG 92

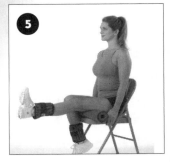

Seated Leg Extension   PG 88

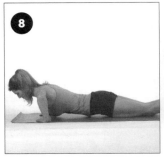

Pigeon Push-Ups   PG 91

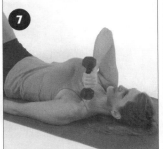

Lying Tricep Crossover   PG 90

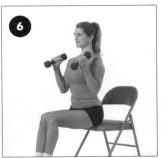

Seated Hammer Curls   PG 89

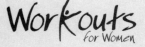

Knee Up / Curl Back Combo

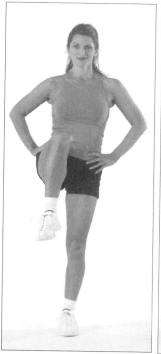 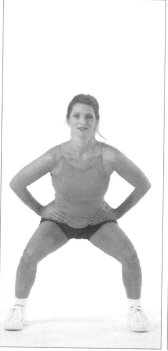 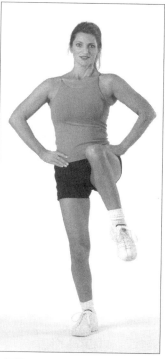

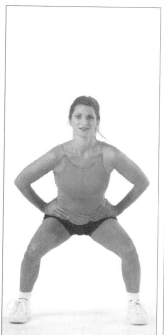 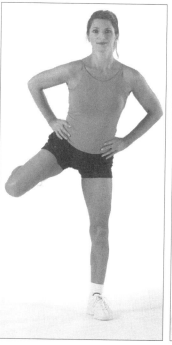 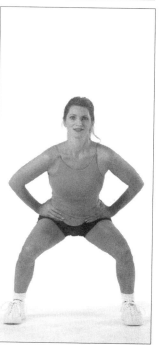

SET UP

Stand tall with shoulders back, chest high and abdomen held in tight, with hands on your waist. Legs should be outside shoulder width apart with knees soft.

TIPS FROM JONI

Increase the intensity of this move by adding in arm movements.

Circuit Seven

Knee Up / Curl Back Combo (continued)

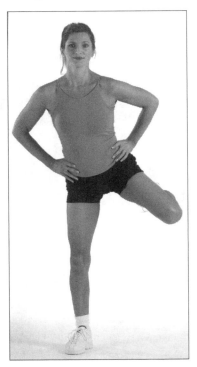 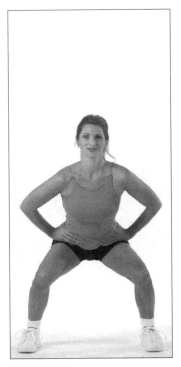

Exercise Technique

1. Bring one knee up to your chest.

2. Lower the leg and bring the opposite knee up to your chest.

3. Curl the opposite leg up and back, bringing the foot up toward your buttocks.

REPEAT THE CURL UP WITH THE OPPOSITE LEG.

ALTERNATE BETWEEN KNEE-UPS AND CURL-BACKS FOR 2 MINUTES.

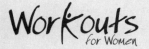

Rotate-in Overhead Press

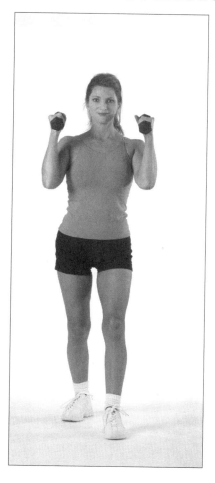 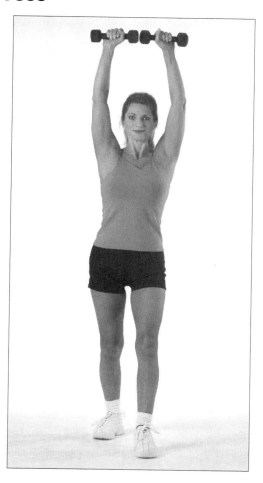

SET UP

Stand tall with abdominal muscles held in tight and dumbbells in both hands. Bend arms at the elbows and pull elbows in close to your body with hands at about shoulder height, with palms facing in toward you at shoulder level.

TIPS FROM JONI

When extending arms overhead be sure not to overextend by keeping elbows soft.

Exercise Technique

1. Exhale as you extend your arms straight up overhead, rotating the palms so that they are facing forward at the top.

2. Lower your arms down to start while simultaneously rotating palms in toward each other again.

REPEAT 15 TIMES.

Circuit Seven

Side Lunge

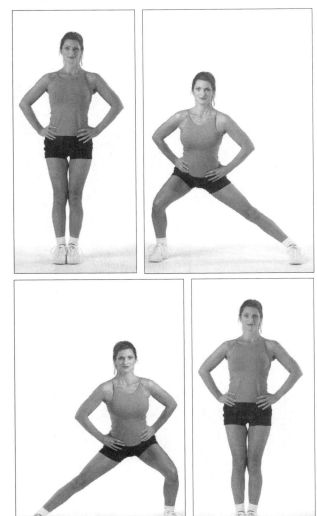

Exercise Technique

1. Take a long step out to the side with one leg, shifting your body weight in the same direction as you bend the knee. Keep the stationary leg straight.

2. Exhale as you press up with the heel and pull the leg back into start.

REPEAT 15 TO 20 TIMES ALTERNATING FROM SIDE TO SIDE.

Squats

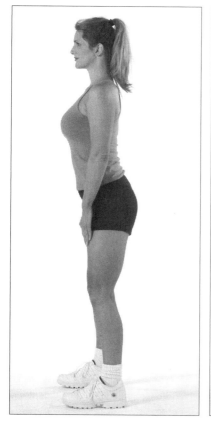 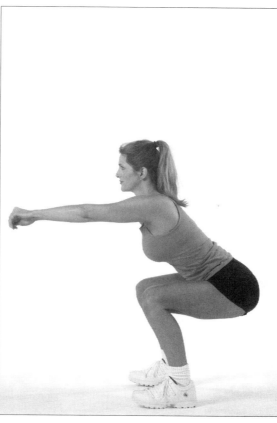

BODY PART WORKED
Buttocks (Gluteal)

SET UP
Stand with feet just outside shoulder width, abdominal muscles held in tight, shoulders back, chest high, and toes pointing straight ahead.

TIPS FROM JONI
Be sure not to allow your knees to extend past your toes as you lower down or you will be placing too much stress on the knees.

Exercise Technique

1. Begin this exercise by bending at the knees, and reach back with your buttocks as if you were sitting on a chair behind you.

2. Stop when your hips are knee level. Do not drop any lower.

3. Exhale as you press yourself back up to standing position with most of your weight pressing up through your heels.

4. Contract the buttocks at the top of the move as you stand back up.

REPEAT 15 TIMES.

BODY PART WORKED
Front of Thighs
(Quadriceps)

SET UP
Sit tall and back on a chair with your abdominal muscles held in tight, shoulders back, and chest high, with an ankle weight around each leg. If necessary, place a rolled-up towel under your knees to raise your legs so that you're touching the floor only with your toes.

TIPS FROM JONI
This exercise is an excellent knee strengthener. If you feel any acute pain in the knees, reduce the amount of weight you are using.

Seated Leg Extension

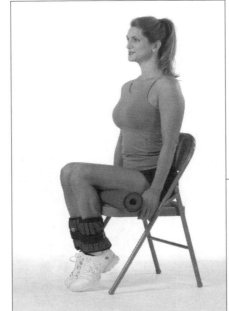

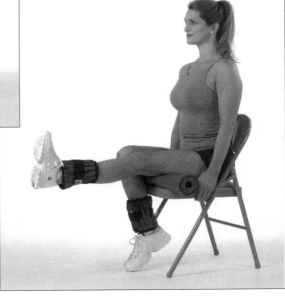

Exercise Technique
1. Flex the foot and exhale as you extend one leg out in front of you, squeezing the thigh muscle in the front of the leg at the top of the move.

2. Bend your knee and lower your leg back down to start.

REPEAT 15 TIMES ON ONE SIDE THEN THE OTHER.

Workouts for Women

Seated Hammer Curls

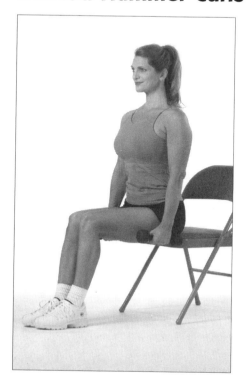 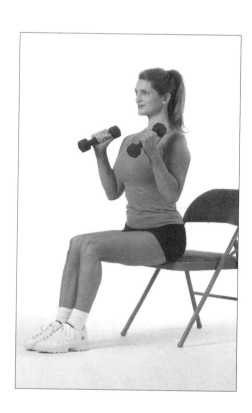

BODY PART WORKED
Front of Arms (Biceps)

SET UP
With dumbbells in each hand, sit tall on the edge of a chair with abdominal muscles held in tight, shoulders back, and chest high. Arms hang down at your sides with palms facing in.

TIPS FROM JONI
Keep elbows stationary at your sides throughout the move, being sure they do not move forward or backward.

Exercise Technique

1. Exhale as you bend your arms at the elbows, lifting hands up toward your shoulders.

2. Extend arms back down to your sides in a controlled manner.

REPEAT 15 TIMES.

BODY PART WORKED

Back Of Arm (Tricep)

SET UP

Lie flat on your back with your knees bent and feet flat on the floor. Hold a dumbbell in one hand and extend it straight up from the shoulder with the palm facing in.

TIPS FROM JONI

Forearms should remain motionless throughout the entire move to be sure to keep the exercise focused and effective for the back of the arm.

Workouts for Women

90

Lying Tricep Crossover

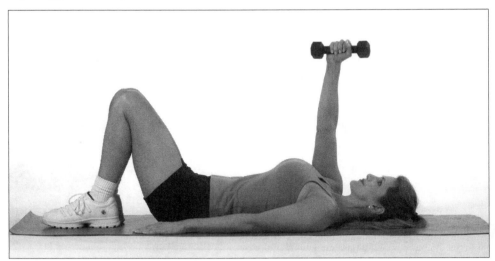

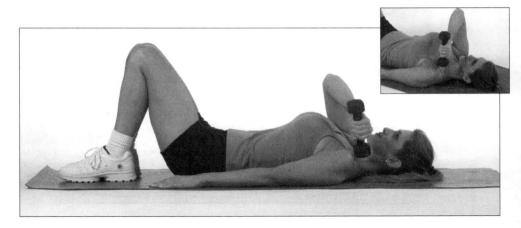

Exercise Technique

1. Keep your upper arm stationary as you bend at the elbow and lower your hand toward the opposite shoulder.

2. Exhale as you extend your arm back up to start, being careful not to lock your elbow at the top of the move.

REPEAT 15 TIMES ON ONE SIDE AND THEN ON THE OTHER.

Pigeon Push-Ups

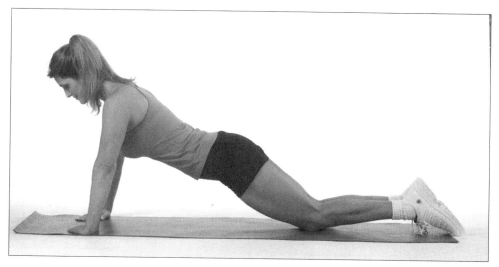

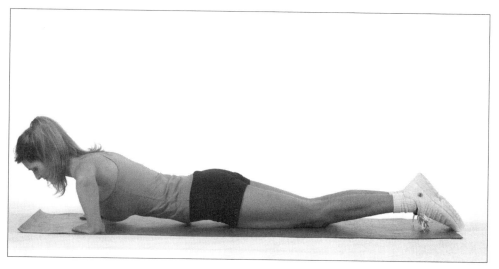

Exercise Technique

1. Bend at the elbows and lower your body toward the floor, stopping when your chest is one fist distance from the floor.

2. Exhale as you push back up to start by straightening your arms.

REPEAT 15 TIMES.

SET UP

Kneel down onto the floor on your hands and knees, with your hands just outside shoulder width apart and fingers pointing in toward each other. Keep your abdominal muscles held in tight.

TIPS FROM JONI

Be careful not to lock your elbows as you push back up to start. Keep your neck in line with your spine throughout the move.

Circuit Seven

BODY PART WORKED

Core Muscles, Including Trunk and Pelvis (Rectus Abdominis and Transverse Abdominis)

SET UP

Lie face down on the floor with your elbows bent right next to your chest resting on your forearms with palms facing down.

TIPS FROM JONI

During the exercise a common tendency is to hold your breath. Be sure to breathe normally throughout the move.

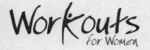

Plank

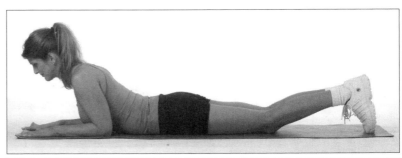

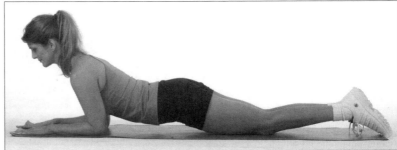

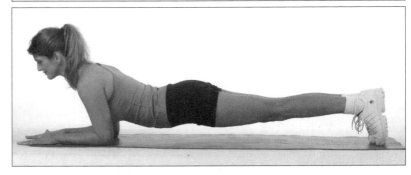

Exercise Technique

1. Exhale as you lift your midsection up off the floor and rise up onto your knees first, then up to your toes and forearms, keeping your back and buttocks flat from knees to shoulders.

2. Hold this position for 15 seconds.

3. Slowly and carefully come back down onto your knees, and move right back into setup position, resting for 5 seconds before lifting up again.

REPEAT THIS MOVE 3 TIMES.

Knee-in Oblique

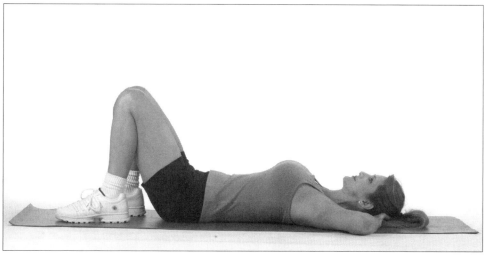

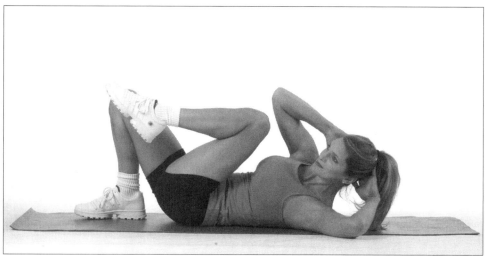

SET UP

Lie on your back with knees bent and heels close to your body. Tilt the pelvis up slightly to flatten out your back. Place fingertips lightly against the back of your head.

TIPS FROM JONI

The lifting and rotating motion really focuses on the waist. Complete each move with precision and focus for maximum results.

Exercise Technique

1. Exhale as you lift and rotate one shoulder toward the opposite knee, as you simultaneously lift that knee toward the shoulder.

2. Lower shoulder and knee back down to start position, then immediately perform the move on the opposite side.

ALTERNATE FROM SIDE TO SIDE FOR A TOTAL OF 20 TO 30 TIMES.

Circuit Seven

EQUIPMENT
Step
Dumbbells

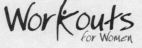

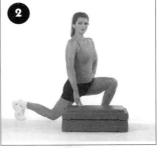

Forward Heel Taps   PG 95

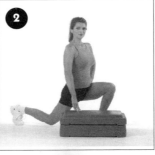

Side Lunge Touch Downs   PG 96

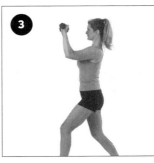

Military Press   PG 97

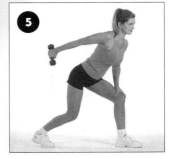

Reach Crunch   PG 104

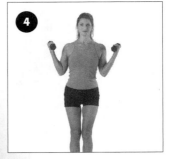

Biceps Curl to the Side   PG 98

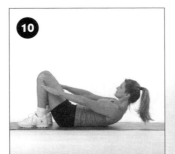

Prone Leg Press   PG 103

Bent-over Triceps Kickback   PG 99

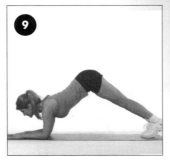

Rotating Chest Press   PG 102

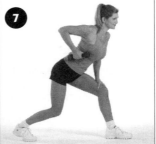

Bent-over Row to Ribs   PG 101

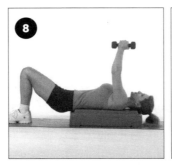
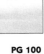

Dead Lift   PG 100

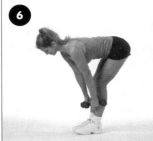

Forward Heel Taps

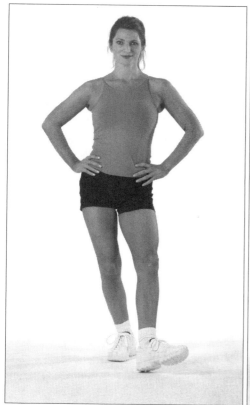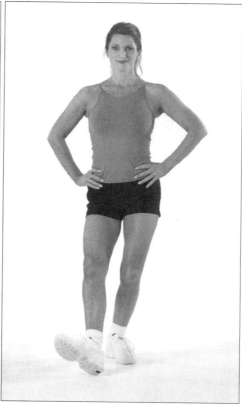

Exercise Technique

1. Tap one heel forward, then the other.

ALTERNATE RIGHT AND LEFT FOR TWO MINUTES.

SET UP
Stand tall with shoulders back, chest high and abdomen held in tight, with hands on your waist. Legs should be outside shoulder width apart with knees soft.

TIPS FROM JONI
Adding in arm movements will increase the intensity of this exercise.

Circuit Eight

Side Lunge Touch Downs

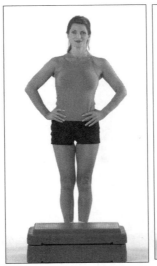 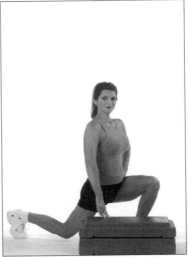 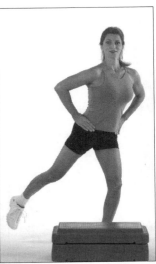

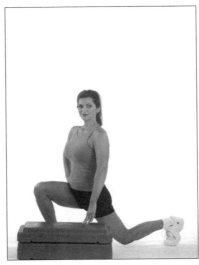 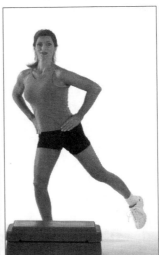 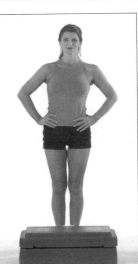

Exercise Technique

1. Extend one leg out to the side, while simultaneously bending the opposite knee as you touch down onto the step with the hand on the same side as the extended leg.

2. Exhale as you pull your extended leg back in and push yourself up with heel of the other leg. Then repeat the move on the other side.

ALTERNATE RIGHT AND LEFT FOR A TOTAL OF 16 TO 20 TIMES.

Military Press

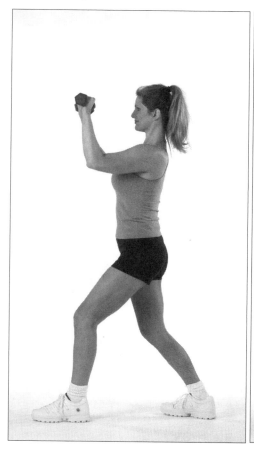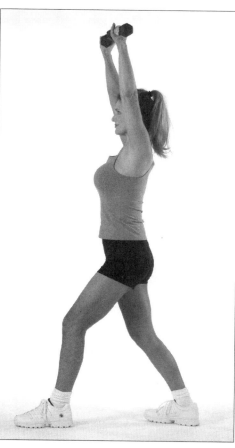

SET UP
Holding dumbbells in both hands, stand tall with abdominal muscles held in tight, shoulders back, and chest high. Start with both arms out in front of your body, bent at the elbows so that hands are shoulder height with palms facing away. Upper arms should be parallel to the floor.

TIPS FROM JONI
Keep elbows pulled in front of your body throughout the move to keep the focus on the front of the shoulders.

Exercise Technique
1. Exhale as you extend arms straight up overhead.

2. Bend at the elbows as you lower back to start.

REPEAT 15 TIMES.

Circuit Eight

97

SET UP

Stand tall with shoulders back, chest high, and abdominal muscles held in tight. Hold dumbbells in each hand. Rest your elbows on the sides of your hips with your arms extended down with palms facing forward.

TIPS FROM JONI

Be sure that elbows remain stationary at your sides throughout the move.

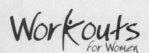

Biceps Curls to the Side

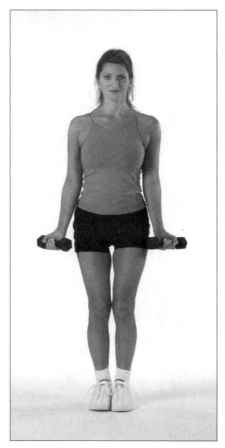
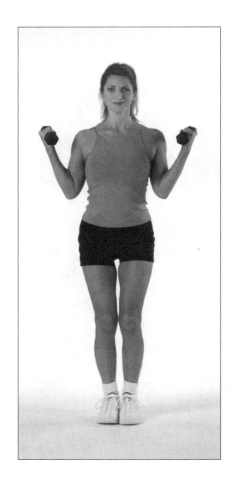

Exercise Technique

1. Exhale as you bend arms at the elbows, bringing hands up toward the sides of your shoulders, with palm facing in toward you at the top of the move.

2. Reverse the motion and extend arms back to start in a controlled manner.

REPEAT 15 TIMES.

Bent-over Triceps Kickback

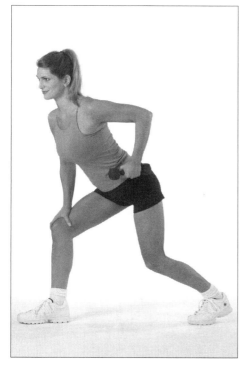

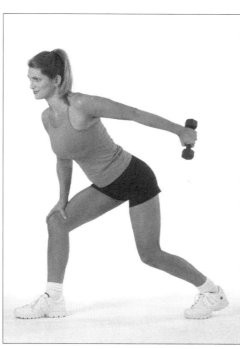

BODY PART WORKED
Back of Upper Arm (Triceps)

SET UP
Begin this exercise in a semi-lunge position, standing with one leg forward and one back. Both knees should be pointing straight ahead, and abdominal muscles should be held in tight. Lean forward, bending at the hip, and rest the forward hand on your forward thigh to support your body. Hold a dumbbell in the other hand and raise the arm up and bend at the elbow, so that the upper arm is in line with your torso and close to your body.

TIPS FROM JONI
Keep your elbow stationary and close to your body throughout the move. Be sure not to swing the working arm. Concentrate on using the muscles in the back of your arm to lift the weight up.

Exercise Technique

1. Exhale as you extend the arm straight back, lifting the weight until your arm is extended straight, feeling the tension in the back of the arm.

2. Lower the arm back to start in a controlled manner.

REPEAT 15 TIMES ON ONE SIDE THEN ON THE OTHER SIDE.

Circuit Eight

BODY PART WORKED

Back of Legs, Lower Back (Hamstring, Erector Spinae)

SET UP

Stand tall with shoulders back, chest high and abdominal muscles held in tight. Position feet loosely together, with dumbbells in hands and arms hanging straight at your sides with palms facing in toward your body.

TIPS FROM JONI

Keep your hands very close to your body throughout the entire move as if you were shaving your legs.

Workouts *for Women*

Dead Lift

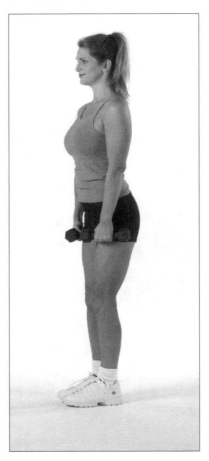 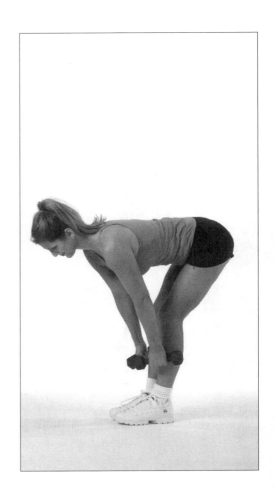

Exercise Technique

1. Keep a slight bend in your knees as you bend forward at the hip, reaching back with your tailbone, allowing your hands to move downward toward your feet.

2. Stop at the point at which you feel slight tension in the back of your legs, then exhale as you stand back up, returning to start.

REPEAT 15 TIMES.

Bent-over Row to Ribs

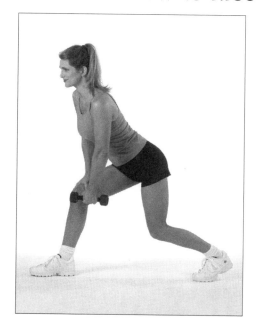

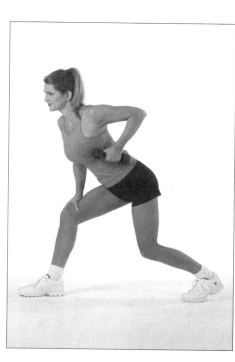

SET UP
Begin this exercise in a semi-lunge position, standing with one leg forward and one back. Both knees should be pointing straight ahead and abdominal muscles should be held in tight. Lean forward bending at the hip, and rest the forward hand on your forward thigh to support your body. Hold a dumbbell in the other hand and position the arm hanging down holding the weight near the forward knee.

TIPS FROM JONI
Be sure to keep your forward hand on the thigh to support your back throughout the move.

Exercise Technique

1. Keeping your hand close to your body, exhale as you lift the weight straight up toward your rib cage, squeezing the shoulder blades together at the top of the movement.

2. Lower the weight back down to start.

REPEAT 15 TIMES ON ONE SIDE THEN ON THE OTHER.

Circuit Eight

SET UP

Lie on a step with your back flat and neck supported. Hold a dumbbell in each hand and bend arms at the elbows so that arms are in a goalpost position with forearms parallel to the floor and with palms facing toward your feet.

TIPS FROM JONI

Keep your wrists straight throughout the move.

Workouts for Women

Rotating Chest Press

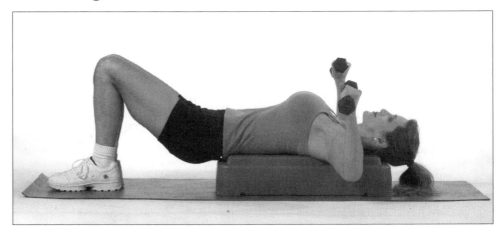

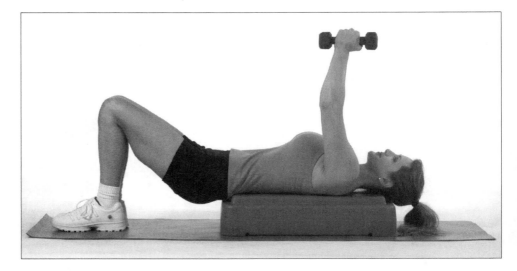

Exercise Technique

1. Exhale as you press the weight up while rotating the palms of your hands in toward each other. Bring hands together at the top of the move.

2. Reverse the move and lower the weight while rotating your hands back out. Stop when your forearms are parallel to the floor.

REPEAT 15 TIMES.

Prone Leg Press

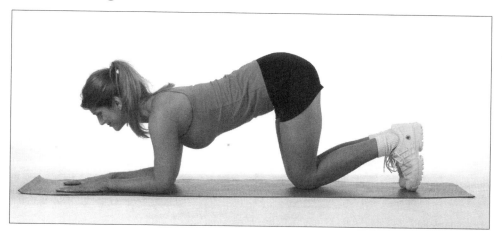

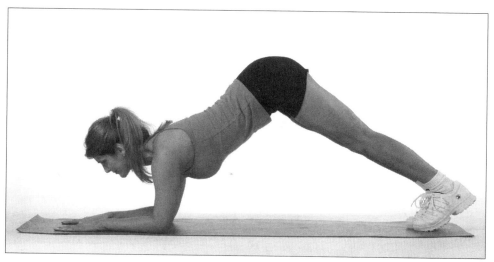

BODY PART WORKED

Front of Thighs (Quadriceps)

SET UP

Kneel down onto your hands and knees with abdomen held in tight. Your knees should be together and directly under your hips and your fingers should be pointing straight ahead.

TIPS FROM JONI

Be sure to maintain proper breathing during this move, since the tendency can be to hold your breath.

Exercise Technique

1. Exhale as you straighten your knees and tighten the fronts of your thighs at the top of the move.

2. Reverse the move and bend at the knees, stopping just before your knees touch back down onto the floor.

REPEAT 15 TIMES.

Circuit Eight

BODY PART WORKED

Upper Abdomen (Rectus Abdominis)

SET UP

Lie flat on your back with your knees bent, heels close to your body, and pelvis tilted slightly upward to help flatten the back. Extend your arms straight overhead.

TIPS FROM JONI

Keep your chin one fist distance off your chest throughout the move.

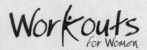

Reach Crunch

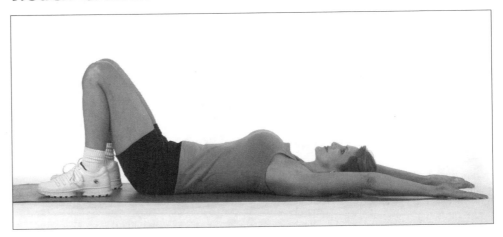

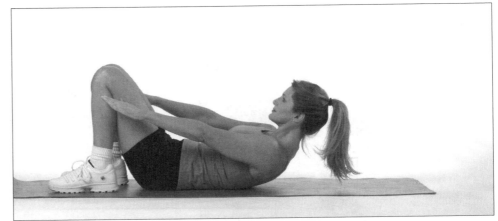

Exercise Technique

1. Exhale as you lift your shoulders and upper back off the floor, bringing your arms moving over your body in an arc reaching forward toward your feet.

2. Reverse the move, lowering your upper back and shoulders toward the floor with your arms extended straight overhead, but not resting your head down on the floor.

REPEAT 20 TO 30 TIMES.

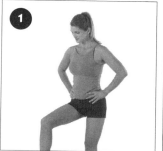
Step Tap on Step **PG 106**

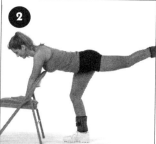
Standing Straight-Leg Glute **PG 107**

Pliés **PG 108**

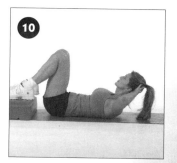
Draped Leg Crunch **PG 115**

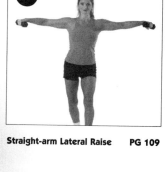
Straight-arm Lateral Raise **PG 109**

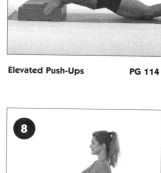
Elevated Push-Ups **PG 114**

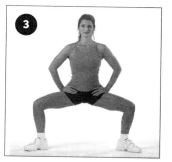
Seated Leg Extension **PG 110**

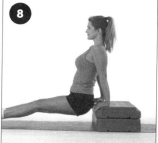
Triceps Dip Off Step **PG 113**

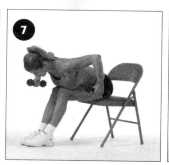
Seated Bent-over Rear Flies **PG 112**

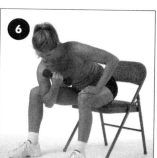
Concentration Curl **PG 111**

EQUIPMENT
Step
Dumbbells
Ankle Weights
Chair

CIRCUIT

Circuit Nine

SET UP

Stand next to the long side of your step with shoulders back, chest high, and abdomen held in tight.

TIPS FROM JONI

To increase the challenge of this exercise, increase the height of the step and/or hold dumbbells in your hands.

Step Tap on Step

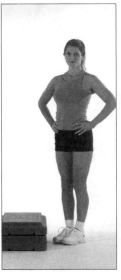 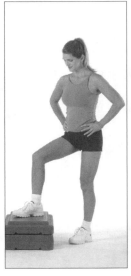 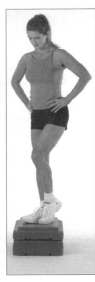 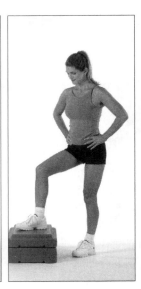

Exercise Technique

1. With the foot closest to the step, step up onto the middle of the step, striking with the heel first.

2. Tap up onto step with the toes of the other foot, then step down onto the floor with that foot followed by the other so you are back to start position standing next to the step.

REPEAT FOR ONE MINUTE ON ONE SIDE, THEN WALK AROUND TO THE OTHER SIDE OF THE STEP AND REPEAT THE MOVE FOR ANOTHER MINUTE.

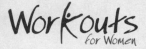

Standing Straight-Leg Glute

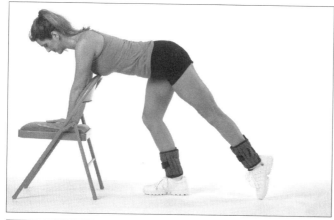

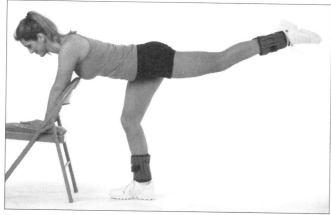

SET UP
Place an ankle weight on each leg. Stand with a slight bend in the knees. Bend forward at the hip and support yourself with your arms leaning onto a chair. Be sure your back is flat and extend one leg straight back with the pointed toes touching the floor.

TIPS FROM JONI
Keep your hips square to the floor at all times.

Exercise Technique
1. Exhale as you lift the extended leg up as high as you can comfortably go. Squeeze the buttocks at the top of the move.

2. Lower the leg back to start, tapping the toe back down to the floor.

REPEAT 15 TIMES ON ONE SIDE THEN 15 TIMES ON THE OTHER.

Circuit Nine

SET UP

Stand with your abdomen held in tight, shoulders back, and chest high, with legs double shoulder width apart. Point your toes out- ward and point your knees in the same direction.

TIPS FROM JONI

To keep the focus of the move on the inner thigh, keep your buttocks tucked under and keep your knees pressing back.

Pliés

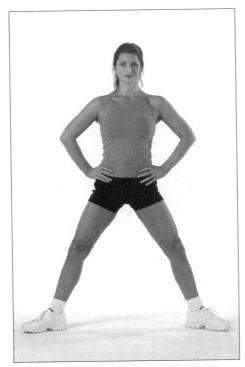
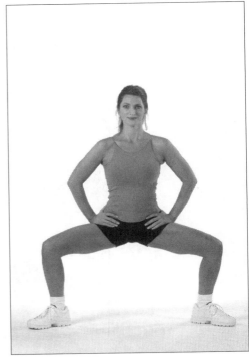

Exercise Technique

1. Bend at the knees, lowering your hips toward the floor, stopping when you feel a stretch in the inner thigh.

2. Exhale and press through your heels, straightening your legs returning back to start.

REPEAT 15 TIMES.

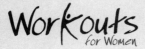

Straight-arm Lateral Raise

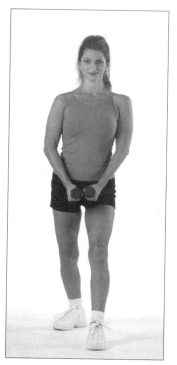 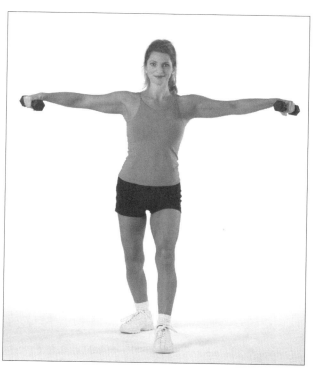

SET UP
Stand tall with feet together and knees slightly bent, with shoulders back, chest high, and abdomen held in tight. Hold dumbbells in each hand with arms hanging down in front of your body with palms facing in toward each other.

TIPS FROM JONI
At the top of the move check for proper form being sure that hands and elbows are at the same height and that your wrists are straight.

Exercise Technique

1. Keep arms straight and exhale as you lift arms directly out to the side, stopping at shoulder height.

2. Control the resistance as you lower your arms back down to starting position.

REPEAT 15 TIMES.

Circuit Nine

SET UP

Sit tall and back on a chair with your abdominal muscles held in tight, shoulders back, and chest high with an ankle weight around each leg. If necessary, place a rolled-up towel under your knees to raise your legs so that you're touching the floor only with your toes.

TIPS FROM JONI

This exercise is an excellent knee strengthener. If you feel any acute pain in the knees, reduce the amount of weight you are using.

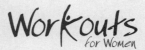

Seated Leg Extension

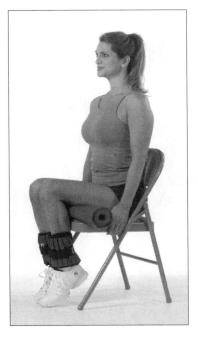 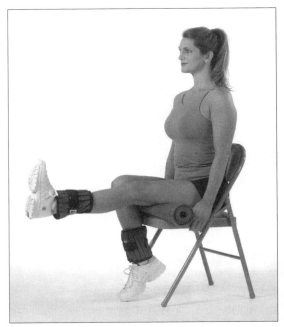

Exercise Technique

1. Exhale and flex the foot and extend one leg out in front of you, squeezing the thigh muscle in the front of the leg at the top of the move.

2. Bend your knee and lower your leg back down to start.

REPEAT 15 TIMES ON ONE SIDE THEN THE OTHER.

Concentration Curl

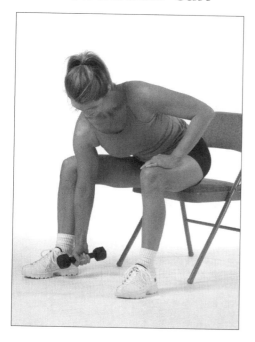 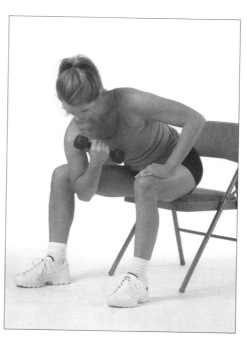

Exercise Technique

1. Keep your elbow in place and extend the arm, lowering the weight until your arm is hanging straight down.

2. Exhale as you curl the weight back up in an arc toward the shoulder.

REPEAT 15 TIMES ON ONE SIDE, THEN ON THE OTHER.

SET UP
Sit with your buttocks toward the edge of a chair, holding your abdomen in tight with legs a comfortable distance apart. Hold a dumbbell in one hand and rest your elbow on the corresponding thigh. Lean your torso slightly forward toward the knee of the working arm and place the other hand on the opposite thigh for support.

TIPS FROM JONI
Keep your back straight. Do not allow it to arch.

Circuit Nine

Workouts for Women

Seated Bent-over Rear Flies

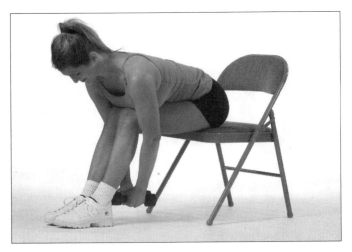

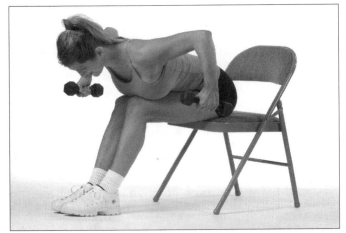

Exercise Technique
1. Exhale as you bend arms at the elbows and pull your hands up toward the rib cage, squeezing your shoulder blades together at the top of the move.

2. Reverse the move and lower your arms back to start in a controlled manner.

REPEAT 15 TIMES.

Triceps Dip Off Step

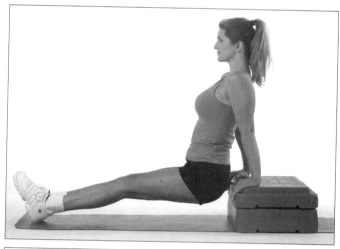

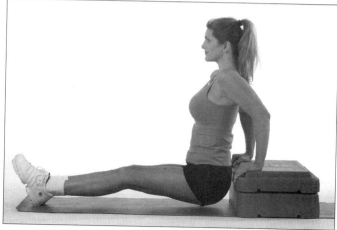

SET UP
Sit on the long edge of a step with your hands gripping the edge. Extend your legs out straight. Move your buttocks off the step and extend your arms straight.

TIPS FROM JONI
Keep your buttocks close to the step throughout the move.

Exercise Technique

1. Bend your elbows directly behind you, lowering your hips toward the floor, stopping before you feel any pressure in your shoulders.

2. Exhale as you push back up to start until elbows are almost straight.

REPEAT 15 TIMES.

Circuit Nine

SET UP

Kneel down on the floor on your hands and knees behind the long side of your step. Grip the edge of the step with your hands just outside shoulder width apart.

TIPS FROM JONI

Be careful not to lock your elbows as you push back up to start. Keep your abdominal muscles tight and your neck in line with your spine throughout the move.

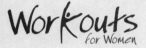

Elevated Push-Ups

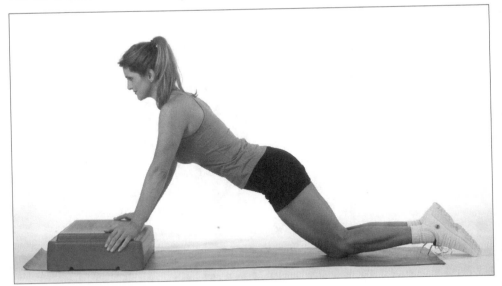

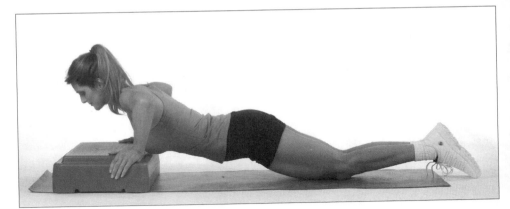

Exercise Technique

1. Bend at the elbows and lower your body toward the step. Stop when your chest is one fist distance from the step.

2. Exhale as you push back up to start by straightening your arms.

REPEAT 15 TIMES.

Draped Leg Crunch

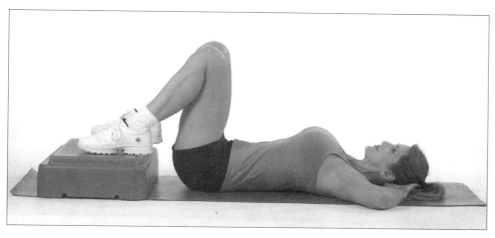

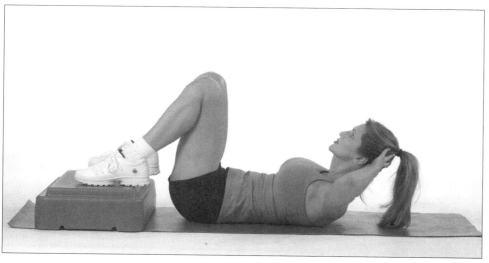

Exercise Technique

1. Exhale as you lift your shoulders and upper back off the floor, moving your rib cage toward your hips.

2. Reverse the move, lowering your upper back and shoulders toward the floor, but not resting your head down onto the floor.

REPEAT 15 TO 20 TIMES.

BODY PART WORKED
Upper Abdomen (Rectus Abdominis)

SET UP
Lie flat on your back behind the long end of your step with your feet on top. Place your fingertip lightly against the back of your head.

TIPS FROM JONI
Keep your chin one fist distance off your chest throughout the move.

TEN

CIRCUIT

EQUIPMENT

Step
Dumbbells
Ankle Weights
Chair

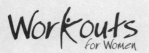

Workouts *for Women*

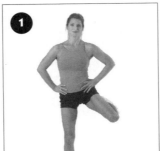

1 Curl Backs PG 117

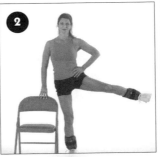

2 Standing Outer Thigh PG 118

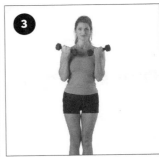

3 Biceps Curls PG 119

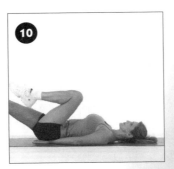

10 Bicycles PG 126

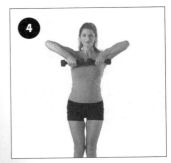

4 Upright Row PG 120

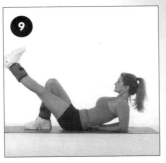

9 Seated Leg Press PG 125

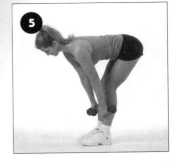

5 Dead Lift PG 121

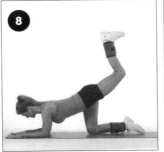

8 Mule Pulses PG 124

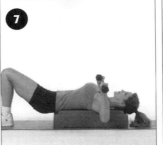
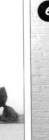

7 End-to-End Chest Press on Step PG 123

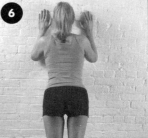

6 Triceps Wall Pushups PG 122

Curl Backs

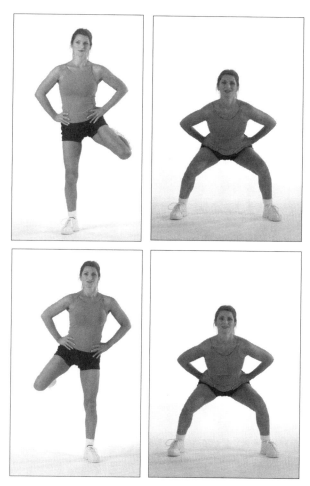

SET UP
Stand tall with shoulders back, chest high, and abdomen held in tight, with hands on your waist. Legs should be outside shoulder width apart with knees soft.

TIPS FROM JONI
Increase the intensity of this move by adding in arm movements.

Exercise Technique

1. Curl one leg up, bending at the knee and bringing the foot up toward your buttocks, shifting your body weight onto the other leg.

2. Lower the leg down and curl the opposite foot up toward the buttocks shifting your body weight onto the opposite foot.

ALTERNATE FROM SIDE TO SIDE FOR 2 MINUTES.

Circuit Ten

SET UP

With an ankle weight around each leg, stand next to a chair with a slight bend in the knees holding onto the chair for balance. Hold abdomen in tight, chest high and shoulders back.

TIPS FROM JONI

Keeping the toes rotated forward forces you to lift with the heel and keeps the focus of this exercise on the outer thigh.

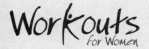

Standing Outer Thigh

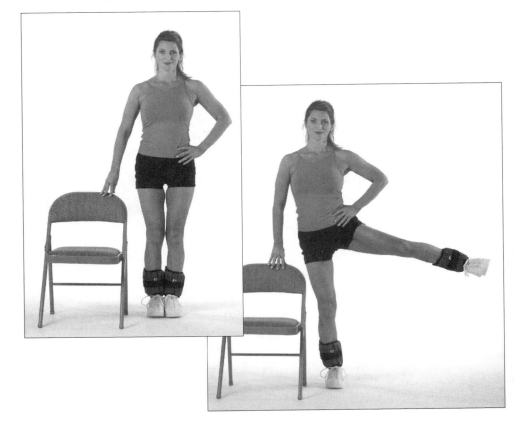

Exercise Technique

1. Begin with the leg that is away from the chair. Rotate the toes inward toward your body. Keeping the toes rotated inward, lead with the heel and exhale as you lift the leg directly out to the side up as far as you can comfortably go without moving your hips.

2. Lower the leg back down to start in a controlled manner, grazing the floor with your foot but not resting it before you lift again.

REPEAT 15 TIMES, THEN MOVE TO THE OTHER SIDE OF THE CHAIR AND REPEAT WITH THE OTHER LEG.

Biceps Curls

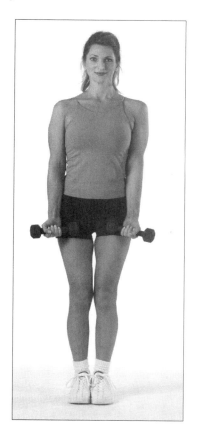 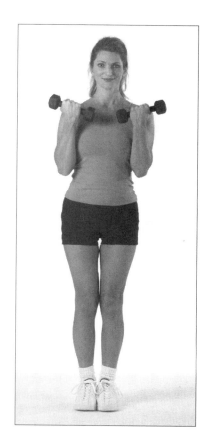

BODY PART WORKED
Front of Arms (Biceps)

SET UP
Stand tall with shoulders back, chest high, and abdomen held in tight. Place arms down at your sides holding dumbbells in each hand with palms of your hands facing forward.

TIPS FROM JONI
Be sure not to rock your body as you lift. This will cause you to use momentum to lift the weight rather than your arm muscles.

Exercise Technique

1. Keeping your elbows stationary, exhale as you bend at the elbows, lifting the weight up toward your shoulders.

2. In a controlled manner, lower your arms back down to start position.

REPEAT 15 TIMES.

Circuit Ten

BODY PART WORKED

Shoulders (Medial Deltoid)

SET UP

With a dumbbell in each hand stand tall with shoulders back, chest high, and abdomen held in tight with palms facing in right in front of your thighs.

TIPS FROM JONI

Keep your hands very close to your body throughout the move.

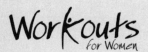

Upright Row

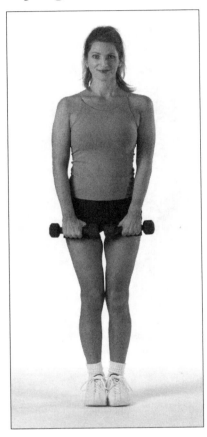
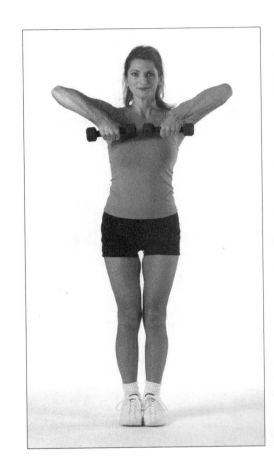

Exercise Technique

1. Bend your elbows up and out to the sides pulling the weight upward, stopping when elbows are shoulder level.

2. Reverse the move and extend your arms back down to start.

REPEAT 15 TIMES.

Dead Lift

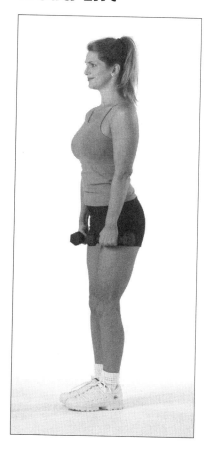

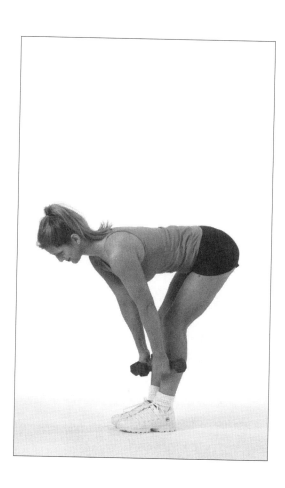

Exercise Technique

1. Keep a slight bend in your knees as you bend forward at the hip, reaching back with your tailbone, allowing your hands to move downward toward your feet.

2. Stop at the point at which you feel slight tension in the back of your legs, then exhale as you stand back up returning to start.

REPEAT 15 TIMES.

Circuit Ten

SET UP

Stand about a foot and a half away facing a wall. Place your hands flat on the wall shoulder width apart and at shoulder height.

TIPS FROM JONI

Keep your elbows pulled in close to your body throughout the move to keep the focus on the back of the arms.

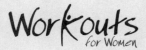

Triceps Wall Pushups

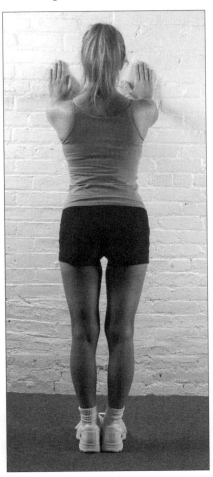
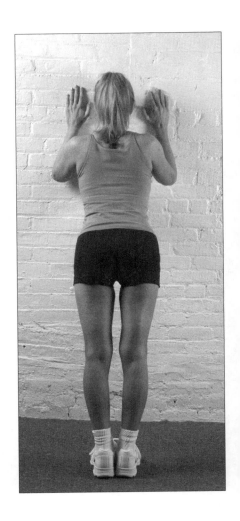

Exercise Technique

1. Bend your elbows until your chest is a few inches from the wall.

2. Exhale as you push with your hands back to start position.

REPEAT 15 TIMES.

End-to-End Chest Press on Step

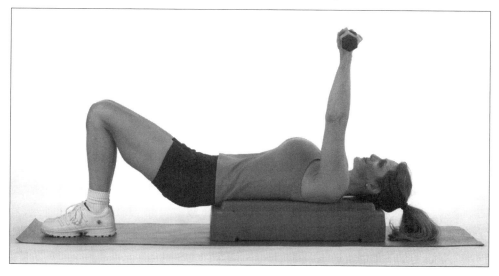

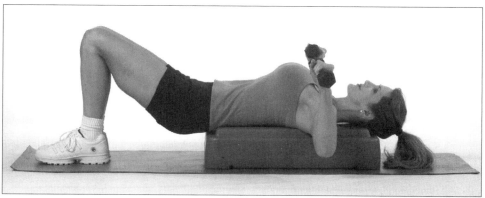

Exercise Technique

1. Bend at the elbows as you lower the weight straight downward, stopping when you feel a stretch through the chest.

2. Exhale as you extend your arms, pressing the weight straight back up to start.

REPEAT 15 TIMES.

BODY PART WORKED
Chest (Pectoral)

SET UP
Lie on a step with your back flat and neck supported. Hold a dumbbell in each hand and extend both arms straight up from your shoulders in line with your chest, with palms facing away from you.

TIPS FROM JONI
Keep your wrists straight throughout the move.

Circuit Ten

123

TIPS FROM JONI
Keep your neck in a relaxed position. Keep both hips square to the ground during the entire movement.

Workouts for Women

Mule Pulses

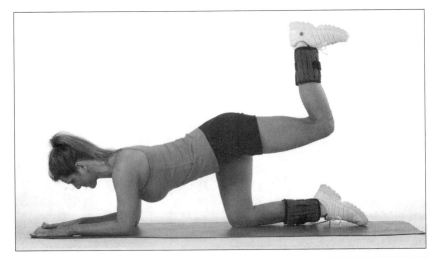

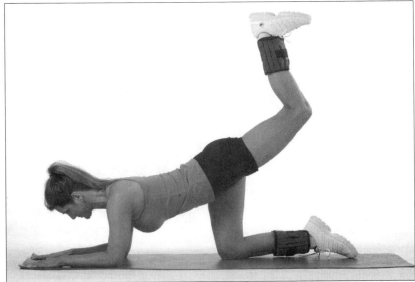

Exercise Technique

1. Pulse (tiny upward movement) the leg up from starting position, squeezing the buttocks at the top of the move.

REPEAT 15 TIMES ON ONE SIDE THEN 15 ON THE OTHER.

Seated Leg Press

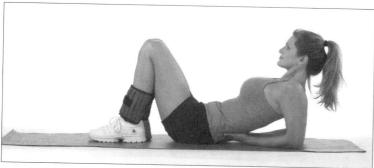

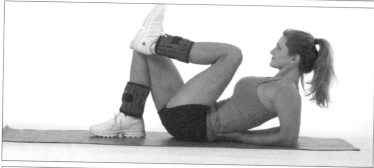

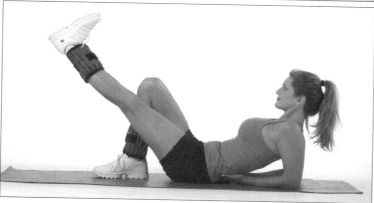

SET UP
With an ankle weight on each leg, sit down on the floor, propping yourself up by placing your hands on your lower back with fingertips pointing toward feet, leaning on your forearms. Bend both legs at the knees and place your feet flat on the floor.

TIPS FROM JONI
Keep your foot at the same height as your knee throughout the move.

Exercise Technique

1. Keeping the knee bent, lift one leg up to a 90-degree angle so that lower leg is parallel to the floor. Flex your foot by pulling your toes in toward you.

2. Leading with the heel, exhale as you extend the leg out.

3. Bend the knee, pulling back to start.

REPEAT 15 SIDES ON ONE SIDE THEN 15 ON THE OTHER.

Circuit Ten

BODY PART WORKED

Lower Abdomen (Rectus Abdominis)

SET UP

Lie on your back with hands palms down underneath buttocks to lift the pelvis up slightly and flatten the back. Lift both legs up with knees bent to a 90-degree angle.

TIPS FROM JONI

Concentrate on using your abdominal muscles to perform this move and not momentum.

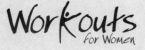

Bicycles

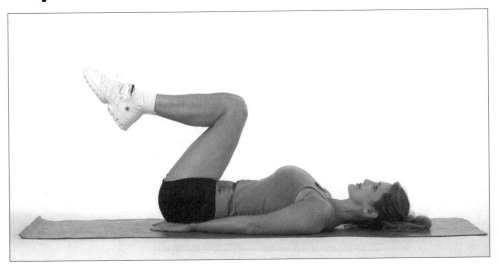

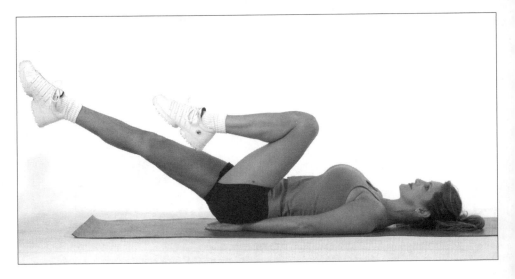

Exercise Technique

1. Exhale as you extend one leg out straight and parallel to the floor, as opposite knee simultaneously bends and comes in toward chest.

ALTERNATE FROM SIDE TO SIDE, REPEATING 20 TO 30 TIMES.

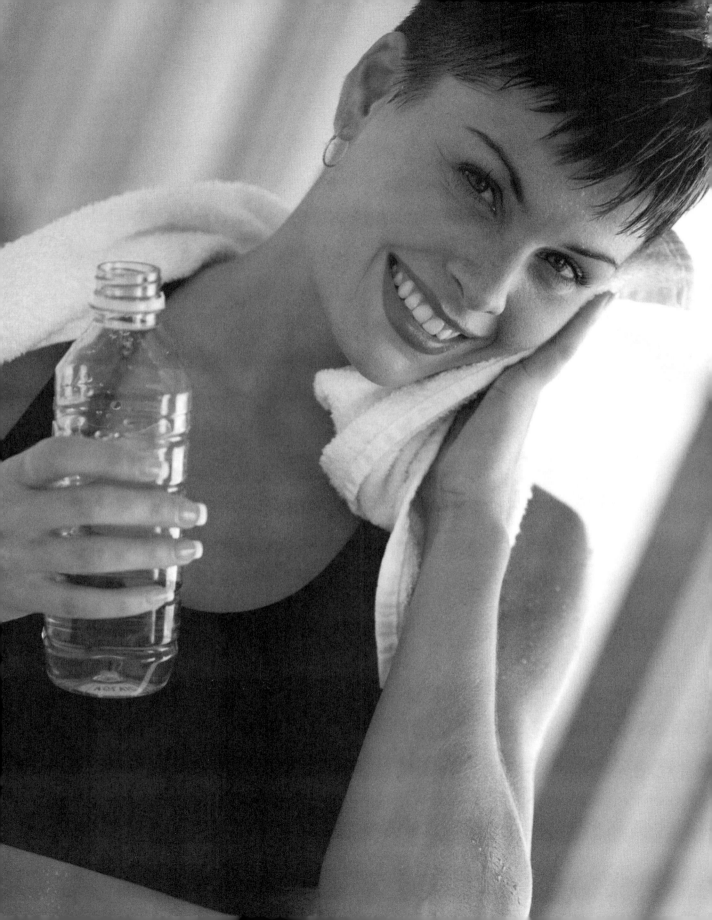

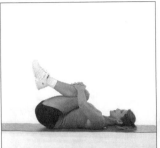
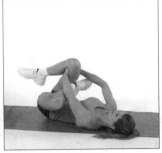
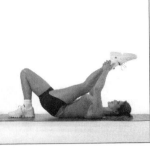

Lower Back Stretch　　　**PG 129**　　　**Hips and Buttocks Stretch**　　　**PG 130**　　　**Back-of-Leg Stretch**　　　**PG 130**

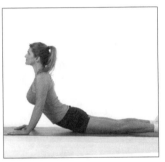
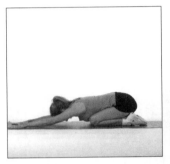

Abdominal Stretch　　　**PG 131**　　　**Shoulder Stretch**　　　**PG 131**

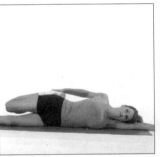
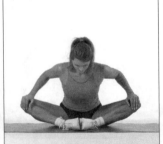
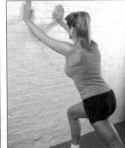

Thigh Stretch　　　**PG 132**　　　**Inner Thigh Stretch**　　　**PG 132**　　　**Calf Stretch**　　　**PG 133**

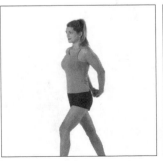
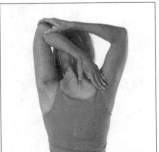
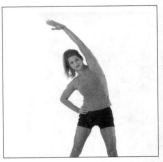

Chest Stretch　　　**PG 133**　　　**Back-of-Arm Stretch**　　　**PG 134**　　　**Torso Stretch**　　　**PG 135**

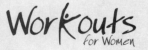
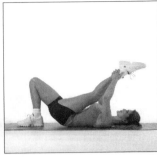

wer Back Stretch

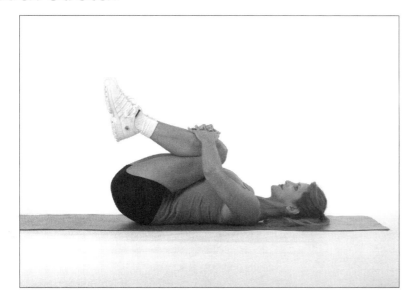

rcise Technique

Lie on your back with both knees bent and feet flat onto the floor.

Keeping your feet and knees together, lift your feet off the floor.

Clasp hands on top of knees, hugging your knees in toward your chest, while keeping your back flat to the floor.

Hold the stretch at the point that you feel mild tension in your lower back.

Hip and Buttocks Stretch

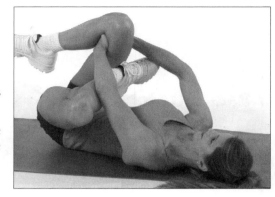

Exercise Technique

1. Lie on your back with your knees bent and feet flat on the floor.

2. Lift one leg up and position the ankle on top of the opposite thigh, just below the knee.

3. Reach around the opposite leg with both hands.

4. Gently pull your knee up and towards your body.

5. Hold the stretch at the point that you feel mild tension in the hip and buttock of the leg that is resting on the thigh. Repeat on the other side.

Back-of-Leg Stretch

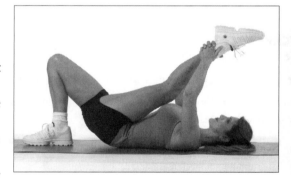

Exercise Technique

1. Lie on your back with knees bent and feet flat on the floor.

2. Lift one leg up, keeping the knee slightly bent and foot flexed.

3. Clasp ankle of lifted leg with both hands.

4. Gently pull your leg towards your body.

5. Hold the stretch at the point that you feel mild tension in the back of the lifted leg.

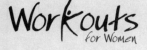

Abdominal Stretch

Exercise Technique

1. Lie face down on the floor.

2. Position your hands directly under shoulders. Point your toes.

3. Exhale as you extend your arms straight, which will lift your chest and abdomen up off the floor.

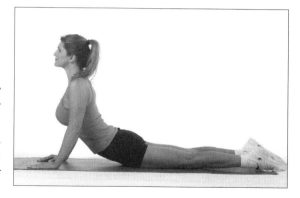

4. Hold the stretch when you feel mild tension through the abdominal muscles.

Shoulder Stretch

Exercise Technique

1. Kneel down on the floor on your hands and knees.

2. Sit back, moving your buttocks toward your heels with your arms extending out in front of your body. Keep your elbows straight and press palms down onto the floor.

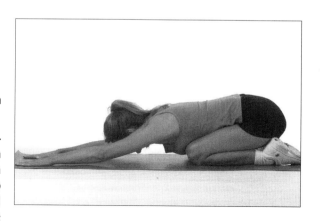

3. Hold the stretch at the point that you feel mild tension through upper arms and shoulders.

MUSCLE STRETCHED
Deltoids

Thigh Stretch

Exercise Technique

1. Lie face down on the floor.

2. Position your hands directly under shoulders. Point your toes.

3. Exhale as you extend your arms straight, which will lift your chest and abdomen up off the floor.

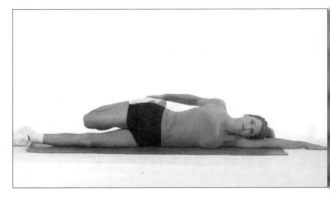

4. Hold the stretch when you feel mild tension through the abdominal muscles.

Inner Thigh Stretch

Exercise Technique

1. Sit tall on the floor with your knees bent and with the bottom of your feet together.

2. Bring your feet in toward your body.

3. Place your hands on your knees and lean your chest forward as you gently press downward on your knees.

4. Hold the stretch at the point that you feel mild tension in your inner thighs.

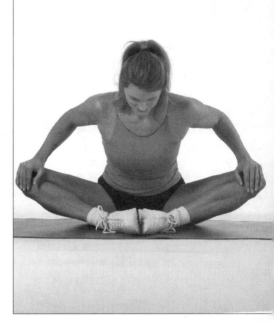

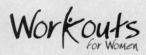

Calf Stretch

Exercise Technique

1. Face a wall, standing about 12 inches away.

2. Place your forearms against the wall and lean forward.

3. Step back with one leg and press the heel down.

4. Hold the stretch at the point that you feel mild tension in the back of the lower part of the extended leg.

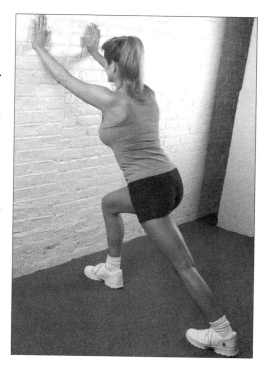

Chest Stretch

Exercise Technique

1. Reach behind your back and clasp fingers together as you lift the chest upward.

2. Hold the stretch at the point that you feel mild tension through the chest.

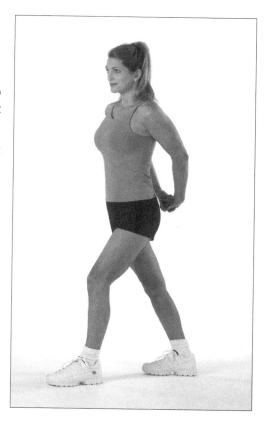

MUSCLE STRETCHED

Pectoral

Stretch Routine

Back-of-Arm Stretch

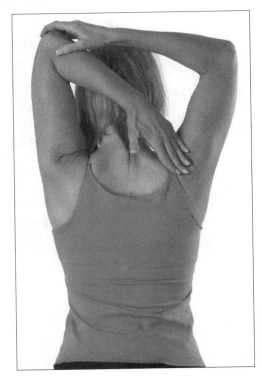

Exercise Technique

1. Stand tall. Drop your chin down toward your chest.

2. Reach one arm straight up overhead with the palm of your hand facing forward.

3. Bend your arm at the elbow and drop your hand to the back of your neck with your palm facing in.

4. Reach overhead with the opposite arm and grasp the arm just below the elbow.

5. Gently pull the elbow in toward the center of your head.

6. Hold the stretch at the point that you feel mild tension in the back of the upper arm. Repeat on the other side.

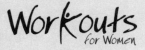

Torso Stretch

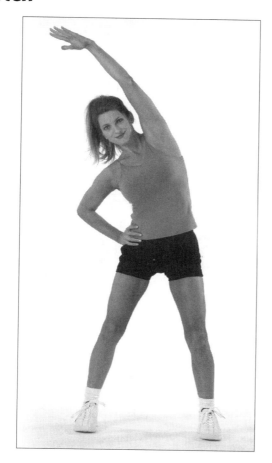

Exercise Technique

1. Stand with your feet just outside shoulder width with toes pointing straight ahead.

2. Place one hand on the hip for support.

3. With the opposite arm reach overhead, bending your torso to the side.

4. Hold the stretch at the point that you feel mild tension through your torso. Repeat on the other side.

Stretch Routine

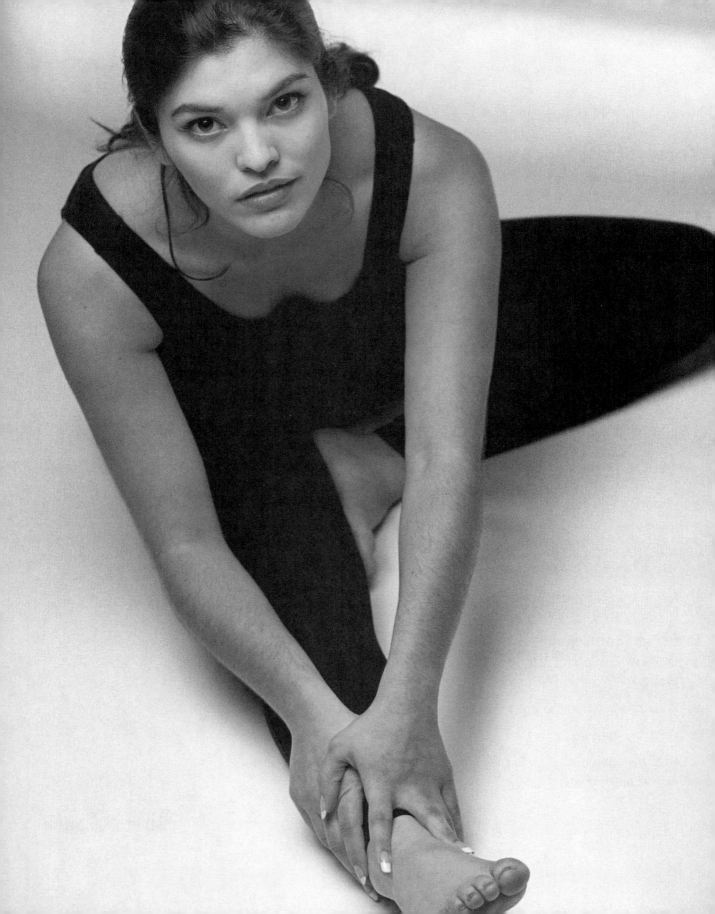

Part
3

Putting It Together

Healthy Eating Plan

Mini-Meals For Long-Term Weight Control

Research has shown that eating five or six smaller meals (mini-meals) has substantial benefits that you do not receive when only eating the traditional three squares. So the first step to weight loss and long-term weight control is to adopt a regular meal pattern of eating smaller mini-meals throughout the day.

A healthy mini-meal consists of 150 to 400 calories and contains a healthy balance of carbohydrates, fats and protein. Here are three main benefits of eating mini-meals:

You will burn up to 10 percent more calories a day. This is due to the thermal effect of feeding which is more active when you eat smaller meals more often, rather than fewer larger meals.

You will put less stress on your heart. Eating a big meal can increase an individual's risk of having a heart attack. A heavy meal makes the heart beat up to 30% faster. Smaller meals lessen this effect.

You will stabilize your blood sugar. Eating healthy mini-meals can help stabilize blood sugar, which will help you stave off cravings, mood swings, and headaches, which are sometimes caused by insulin surges.

Three-Day Mini-Meal Plan

This meal plan is designed to promote weight loss in healthy individuals. This advice should not replace or take precedence over the advice of your health care provider. Please consult with your health care provider before beginning this meal plan and follow his or her recommendation.

Healthy eating and exercise go hand in hand. To maximize your energy level while exercising and to ensure that your metabolism is running efficiently, proper nutrition through balanced meals is essential. This three-day meal plan features the following:

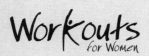

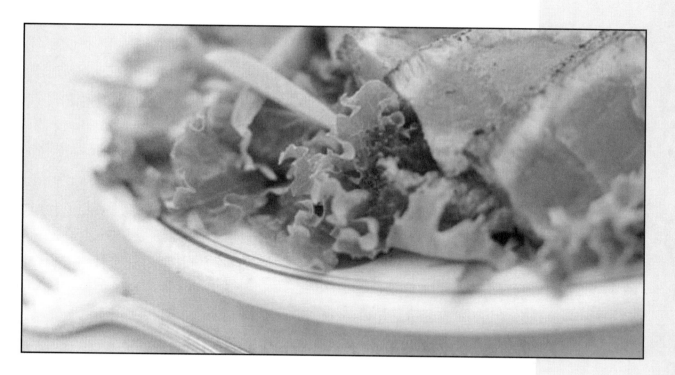

- Carbohydrates with low to moderate glycemic index values to raise blood sugar levels gradually, reducing the production of the fat-storing hormone insulin.

- Five small meals each day, which research has shown to be healthier and more beneficial than the traditional three larger meals.

- Mini-meals that are approximately 400 calories, with snacks of approximately 150 calories to maintain a caloric intake of 1,500 calories per day.

- Small frequent meals that are high in fiber to promote weight loss, lower cholesterol levels, and stabilize blood sugar levels.

- Mini-meals that include a variety of fresh produce and herbs, creating meals high in phytonutrients, which are key to maintaining optimal health.

- Mini-meals that emphasize a diet low in processed foods and refined sugars. Included are whole grains and plentiful servings of fresh fruits, vegetables, and high biological value proteins to maximize the amount of nutrients per meal.

- Evenly spaced meals throughout the day to keep your appetite satisfied.

Healthy Eating Plan

Day 1

Breakfast
MORNING PARFAIT

1 cup sliced strawberries

1 cup low-fat vanilla yogurt

1/2 cup granola

Layer strawberries, yogurt and granola in stemmed parfait glass.

Snack
CHEESY QUESADILLAS

2 whole wheat tortillas

1 oz. grated jack cheese

1 Tbsp. lite sour cream

1 Tbsp. red bell pepper, diced

Sprinkle cheese on one tortilla and cover with second tortilla. Place on plate and microwave for 30 seconds. Cut into wedges and garnish with sour cream and peppers.

Lunch
CHICKPEA-TA POCKETS

1/2 cup canned garbanzo beans, drained and rinsed

1/2 cup fresh spinach, shredded

1/2 cup seedless grapes, halved

1/4 cup red bell pepper, finely chopped

1/4 cup celery, thinly sliced

1/4 cup red onion, finely chopped

1/4 cup lite mayonnaise

2 Tbsp. poppy seed salad dressing

1 pita round, cut in half

In a large bowl combine garbanzo beans, spinach, grapes, pepper, celery and onion. In a small bowl stir together mayo and poppy seed dressing. Add to garbanzo bean mixture. Spoon into pita halves.

Snack
PEAR WITH ALMONDS

1/2 medium bartlett pear

1 Tbsp. dry roasted almonds

Dinner
HAWAIIAN STIR FRY

1 Tbsp. garlic butter

1 12-oz. bag fresh stir-fry veggies

1/2 cup water

1/4 cup teriyaki sauce

1 cup fresh pineapple chunks

1/2 cup whole grain brown rice, cooked

1/4 cup macadamia nuts, crushed

Melt garlic butter in wok or large sauté pan on media high heat. Add veggies and stir for 3 minutes. Add water, teriyaki and pineapple and cook for 7–8 minutes. Mix nuts and rice on the side.

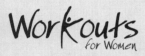

Workouts for Women

Day 2

Breakfast
BROCCOLI AND CHEDDAR QUICHE

1 cup broccoli, chopped

2 whole eggs

2 egg whites

1/4 cup part-skim mozzarella cheese, grated

2 Tbsp. evaporated skim milk

8 oz. vegetable juice

Microwave broccoli for 2 min. Wisk whites, whole eggs and evaporated milk. When blended, add cheese and broccoli into mix and pour into dish. Bake for 20-30 minutes at 350° F.

Snack
SWEET POTATO SKINS

1 sweet potato, baked with skin

4 Tbsp. part skim mozzarella cheese

1/2 cup broccoli, chopped

2 Tbsp. chives

Slice baked potato in half lengthwise and scoop out pulp. Fill skins with broccoli and cheese. Sprinkle chives on top. Bake skins for approx. 15 minutes at 450° F.

Lunch
FRUITY CHICKEN WRAP

3 oz. boneless, skinless chicken breast

1 Tbsp. fat-free ranch dressing

1/4 cup peach or pear slices, drained and chopped

1/4 cup canned mandarin oranges, drained

1/4 cup diced red or green bell peppers

1 green onion, chopped

1/3 cup lite mayonnaise

2 Tbsp. lime juice

dash cayenne pepper

1 whole-wheat tortilla

Arrange chicken breast on broiler pan sprayed with cooking spray. Brush with ranch dressing. Broil at 500° F for 7–10 minutes. Dice chicken. In a bowl, combine chicken, fruit, pepper, and onions. In a separate bowl, stir mayo, lime juice, and cayenne. Add dressing to chicken mixture, spoon onto tortilla, and roll up.

Snack
TOASTED PECANS

1/4 cup pecan halves

1/2 Tbsp. canola oil

Mix pecans with oil and spread evenly onto a microwave-safe dish. Microwave for 1 minute. Stir and microwave for 1 minute intervals until nuts are brown.

Dinner
SPICY KEBOBS AND CORN

2 boneless lean pork chops, cubed

2 Tbsp. taco seasoning

4 scallions, cut into 1" pieces

1/2 green, yellow and red bell peppers, seeded and cut into 1" pieces

1/2 cup corn kernels

Toss pork cubes with seasoning to coat. Thread pork cubes alternately with onion and pepper pieces onto skewers (if using wooden skewers, soak in water 20 min. prior to using). Grill over medium-hot fire, turning until pork is nicely browned, approx. 10 minutes. Heat corn in microwave with 1 Tbsp. of water and serve.

Day 3

Breakfast
BERRY SMOOTHIE

8 oz. fruit-flavored low fat yogurt

1/2 cup crushed Ice

1/2 pumpernickel bagel, toasted

1 Tbsp. butter

Blend smoothie ingredients. Serve with buttered bagel.

Snack
FRESH MELON CUP

1 cup watermelon, cubed

1 cup honeydew melon, cubed

3 Tbsp. lite cool whip

Mix melons in a bowl and top with Cool Whip.

Lunch
CHICKEN RAISIN SALAD

4 oz. grilled ghicken, chopped

1 Tbsp. lite mayonnaise

15 seedless raisins

1/8 cup roasted pistachio nuts, unsalted

2 cups mixed salad greens

3 fresh parsley sprigs

Mix chicken with mayo, raisins, and pistachios. Place on salad greens and garnish with parsley.

Snack
COTTAGE CHEESE
SPRINKLED WITH CASHEWS

1/2 cup low-fat cottage cheese

1 Tbsp. cashews, chopped

Sprinkle cashews on top of cottage cheese.

Dinner
BAKED SALMON
WITH SAFFRON BROWN RICE

5 oz. Atlantic salmon fillet

1 cup long grain brown rice, cooked

1/2 Tbsp. saffron

1 Tbsp. dried rosemary

1 Tbsp. lemon juice

10 fresh bing cherries

Add rosemary and lemon juice on top of salmon fillet and bake at 400° F for 20–30 minutes. Cook brown rice and mix with saffron. Serve cherries on the side.

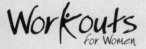

Overcoming Overeating

The uncomfortable feeling experienced after eating too much is something that most of us recognize, but the guilt that goes with it, and the reasons why we do it, are often more difficult to understand. Regular overeating, or out-of-control eating, is eating too often without the prompts of hunger or too much with the promptings of taste. Boredom, stress, and depression are among the reasons why many women habitually overeat—food acts as a source of comfort. Ironically, these "comfort foods" can actually lead to both physical and mental discomfort.

The pattern is the same: You react to an emotional prompt or need by turning to food, but because eating provides only temporary relief, you continue to eat. Having overeaten, you feel bloated, uncomfortable, and guilty about your lack of self-control. These feelings of distress only add to you original stress, and in search of comfort, you end up overeating again!

The key to overcoming overeating is to develop a positive self-image. The first step in this process is to take a good look at your eating patterns so that you can adopt strategies to cope with your overeating triggers. Each success boosts your self-esteem on a daily basis. Only then will you begin to develop a better relationship with your body, your food, and your health.

By their very nature, many diets "deprive" you of certain foods. But when you feel deprived, you may be tempted to overcompensate, eating more then you should. As your weight creeps up again, you feel as though you have failed, and so set even tougher dieting goals. Unable to meet them, you set yet others, and the cycle of failure continues.

Women have appetites for certain foods. When that appetite becomes extreme, it's called a craving. Despite good intentions to eat healthy, cravings can lead you to fatty, sugary, processed carbohydrates and other easy-access snack foods that can in turn, sabotage a healthy lifestyle. But armed with the self-assurance of improved health you can break the shackles of "snacking slavery" by snacking smart.

Be Aware and Be Ready

Cravings can be a result of mood swings or stress, and giving into cravings may serve to mask the symptoms. Address the problem by trying to pinpoint what pushes you into those "snack attack" modes. Notice if your snack attacks happen at a certain time of the month, or certain hour of the day, or if they happen after certain events. Knowing what triggers your cravings is the first step.

SLOW DOWN WHEN YOU EAT

If you're trying to watch your figure, it's a good idea to get in the habit of eating in one place... preferably at the table. You're more likely to overeat when meals are eaten on the run or while you're standing in front of the fridge. Eat slow so you allow your body ample time to let your brain know that you're full.

Healthy Eating Plan

SIMPLE FACTS ABOUT FATS

Every woman needs fat in her diet, but too much of the wrong types of dietary fat is considered a leading cause of heart disease and some cancers, especially breast and colon cancers. Even so, fat is a necessary part of nutrition. It's vital that you know that not all fats are created equal.

Two Types of Fats

Saturated. Most saturated fats come from animal products. The liver converts saturated or hydrogenated fats to cholesterol, which can clog blood vessels. Here are some examples of saturated fats which should be consumed in moderation.

- Pork
- Lamb
- Beef
- Poultry
- Egg Yolk
- Butter
- Milk
- Ice Cream
- Cheese
- Coconut Oil
- Cocoa Butter

Unsaturated. Unsaturated fats include monounsaturated fats and polyunsaturated fats. These hydrogen-light fats may be just as caloric, but they do not block the arteries. In fact, research shows that olive oil and omega-3 polyunsaturated fatty acids found in some cold-water fish may actually help reduce the lipoproteins that transport unhealthy cholesterol.

POLYUNSATURATED
- Corn Oil
- Sunflower Oil
- Soybean Oil
- Cottonseed Oil
- Salmon
- Tuna
- Herring
- Swordfish
- Mackerel
- Walnuts
- Almonds

MONOUNSATURATED
- Olive Oil
- Peanut Oil

When planning your meals, remember that you do need fat in your diet. Many nutritionists recommend that about 20% of your daily caloric intake is from fat and never more than 30%. Choose your fats wisely, opting primarily for the ones that are polyunsaturated and monounsaturated.

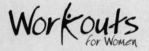

Plan Ahead

Arm yourself and be ready with foods that are good for you to eat close at hand. Stock your pantry and refrigerator with healthy snacks. Whole grain bagels, fresh fruits and vegetables, low-sodium cheeses, low-fat yogurt. Bring naturally sweet fresh fruit, such as grapes or pears, to work with you instead of hitting the vending machine.

Watch Out for the Traps

Certain kinds of trail mixes and granolas may be laden with sugar and fat. Look past labels that say "healthy" or "nutritious" and carefully read the food content. If you normally crave salty foods or meat products, avoid alcohol and sweets. One usually leads to another.

Taking the offense against snack attacks can make all the difference in your weight control program. You can take control, and a little advance planning can make all the difference.

Help for Bingers

If it happens, if you lose control and let all willpower go out the window, it's not time to throw in the towel. Once you're ready to get back in control of your mind and your body, there are a few steps you can take that will put you back on track.

First, prepare to start fresh first thing in the morning. Cleanse your home of all the tempting junk foods. Make a grocery store run and fill your fridge up with healthy snacks. Don't forget to have some of your favorite fruit on hand to ease the sugar withdrawals. Drink lots of water to help cleanse your system. Schedule in exercise time for the upcoming week if you have not already done so, and remember it's not the end of the world. Just a minor setback in the big scheme of things.

Analyze what triggered your binge, what you ate, and where the food came from. With this information clear in your mind, you can develop a strategy for the future. Develop your own plan of how you will avoid situations that lead you to binge and have a plan to follow in place when the urge to binge strikes. Make yourself accountable to someone.

Instead of letting this one nasty slipup become a long-term setback, get right back on the wagon.

Resist the urge to fast the next day. Eat your normal mini-meals, but trim a few hundred calories off your normal daily intake. Also, resist the urge to weigh yourself. Chances are that water retention after your heavy carbohydrate binge will show the scale not to be in your favor. Do you really want to torture yourself like that?

Healthy Eating Plan

Don't go overboard with your workouts or set unrealistic workout goals to compensate for your binge. Just get back onto your normal exercise routine.

Before you give in next time, wait 10 minutes. Then do something to take your mind off of the food. Call a friend, give yourself a pedicure, or take a walk. Also, drink a big cold glass of water.

Remember that you are normal. This happens to everyone from time to time and you have not blown it for good.

Follow these simple steps toward balanced eating and apply them to your daily life.

1. Keep a record of everything you eat for 5 days. Did you go overboard on one food group? Every woman has her own unique tendencies toward diet destruction. Know what yours are.

2. Watch your portions—especially when dining out. When you eat out, take home half for tomorrow's lunch.

3. Stock up on healthy meals at work. Stash goodies such as mini-boxes of raisins in your desk drawer and load the break room fridge with low-fat yogurt, baby carrots, and tomato juice.

4. Plug holes in your diet with healthy snacks. Snack on grapes, veggies, and nuts when you can't sit down and have a mini-meal. You'll be loading up on some very important nutrients and reducing the chance that you'll give in to calorie-laden snacks like chips and cookies.

Food Journals Work

If you're trying to lose weight and adopt healthier eating patterns, keeping track of what you eat by using a food journal can help significantly. A food journal can be a real eye-opener and can help you figure out what changes in your diet you need to focus on.

Researchers say that keeping a food journal allows people to see patterns in their eating. If you have to write it down, you may think twice before having that extra cookie. Furthermore, it works!

Journal-keepers who consistently monitor their food consumption lose weight more steadily (1 to 2 pounds a week) and keep it off. There are several reasons journal-keeping works.

First, when you keep a visual record of what you eat, you can more clearly identify the sources of empty calories.

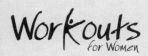

Also, by tracking your activity at the time you ate, you can identify what particular situations prompted you to eat or what time of the day you are most inclined to overindulge in diet-destructive behavior.

For optimal success, it's important to keep your goals in your face all the time. Now is the time to start tracking your eating habits. Keep your journal simple. Remember to total up at the end of the day. (See Appendix II for a sample and blank form.)

Water Works

The average adult woman should drink approximately eight 8-ounce glasses of water a day just to keep up with her body's vital needs. Pregnant women and new mothers require more water than 8 ounces a day, and if you exercise, your body's need for water is also increased. Water serves so many purposes for our bodies. It helps to regulate body temperature, prevents constipation, aids in digestion, helps the body absorb vital nutrients, and curbs appetite. Water replenishes your system and keeps your metabolism running efficiently, especially important while exercising. Water can also be replaced by other beverages including teas, coffee, and non-sugar flavored waters.

Some key tips for making water work for you:

- Drink at least 8 glasses a day—more if you exercise, are pregnant, or are a new mother.
- Flavor water with orange, lemon, or lime slices.
- Have a bottle of water close by you at your desk, in your car or purse.
- Always take water breaks when you are working out.

Calories Count

Yes, it does matter how many calories you consume in a day and over the course of a week. Here's why... It's basic math. Your body needs to store 3,500 calories more than it uses over a period of time for you to gain 1 pound. Likewise, if you use 3,500 calories more than you take in, you will lose 1 pound. Here is a quick formula to help you determine how many calories per pound you need to take in to maintain your current body weight.

First, decide if your activity level is: Low = 12, Moderate =14, or High=16.

Then, multiply the number that corresponds to your activity level by your current weight. The answer is the approximate number of calories you need each day to maintain your current weight.

Healthy Eating Plan

Trying to lose weight? Follow these guideline when crunching calorie numbers.

1. Do not lower caloric intake to less than 1,500 per day or your metabolism may become so slow that your body will work harder to store calories.

2. Expend 300 to 500 calories a day through exercise.

3. Decrease caloric intake to no more than 500 calories below what is necessary to maintain your current weight, then adjust that number as you lose weight.

4. Healthy weight loss is 2 pounds a week... No more!

Set up a reward system for yourself and give yourself a special treat each time you get the job done. One idea is to put a dollar or two in a special tip jar each time you exercise and at the end of the month buy yourself something extra special.

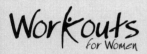

HEALTHY DINING-OUT TIPS

It's a challenge to maintain good eating habits when you eat at restaurants often. Here are some tips that will help you make healthy menu choices when dining out.

1. Start with soup, fruit or raw vegetables, or a light seafood appetizer.

2. Skip the cocktail or limit it to one dry wine or light beer. Sweet wines have about two times the calories. Your best choice: ice water, ice tea, or hot tea.

3. Avoid food that is fried or sautéed.

4. Remove fat from red meats and remove skin from chicken.

5. Avoid rich sauces and dips. Choose red pasta sauces over white.

6. Limit bread to one piece (whole grain is best) and skip the butter or margarine.

7. Avoid crackers, which are usually high in fat and sodium.

8. Order half portions of entrées.

9. Food preparation is important. Choose items that are steamed, broiled, grilled, roasted, baked, or poached.

10. Steer clear of foods that are buttered, fried, creamed, served in gravy, au gratin, scalloped, or rich.

11. Choose a salad bar when possible. Watch out for prepared specialty salads that often contain mayonnaise that is high in fat.

12. Opt for vinegar and oil, lemon juice, or low-fat dressing or buttermilk dressing, rather than regular dressing.

13. For dessert, look for a low-fat option or have a fruit cup or coffee with low-fat cream.

14. Eat slow and stop when you're full.

Healthy
Eating Plan

The Mind-Body Connection

Break Through Internal Barriers

Getting yourself to exercise is 95% mental fortitude and 5% physical. One of the most common reasons women avoid or discontinue their fitness plan is due to internal barriers such as negative thoughts, feelings, and perceptions. You can break through the mental barriers and get your body moving. If you find yourself going through phases of diligent exercise and healthy eating but find it difficult to stick with your plan for very long, it's important that you understand and focus on the benefits of consistent exercise including mental alertness, increased energy, a healthier body, and a physical appearance that you'll be very proud of.

Be realistic and understand the battle ahead. Many women start out their exercise program feeling intimidated, anxious about their appearance, and lacking confidence in their ability to stick with it. Don't let these negative thoughts and feelings stop you from following through with your plans. You CAN do it!

It's also important to establish the right motivation to exercise. True motivation comes from within. Sustain your motivation by setting goals that have personal significance.

Become accountable to a friend or group of women who support you in what you are working toward accomplishing. Statistics tell us that women who are accountable and who receive support are more successful at exercising consistently.

Making It Over a Plateau

Weight-loss plateaus are to be expected, even if you're doing all the right things. When you're in the middle of a plateau, motivation can be hard to come by. Keep reminding yourself that consistent exercise is improving your overall health and fitness, benefiting you on the inside as well as the outside. Also, the psychological benefits can't be beat. Exercise reduces stress levels and anxiety and boosts your self-esteem. Eventually, with consistency, you'll break through that plateau. But in the meantime, here are some things to consider.

1. Maybe you need to be a little pushier. Make sure that your body is challenged during your workouts and if not, consider working out a little longer or a little harder.

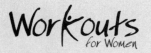

2. Are you eating too many calories? Many women actually underestimate the number of calories they consume. Check your fridge for foods that may be sabotaging your efforts. Be aware of what you eat and how much you eat so you don't negate your exercise efforts.

3. Are you being practical about results? Remember, you didn't gain it in a few weeks. Weight loss takes time and patience.

4. Are you skipping meals? This is a surefire way to slow down your metabolism. Try eating five or six Mini-meals during the day to keep your metabolism working.

5. Are you drinking your results away? Soft drinks, sweetened drinks, and alcohol can mess up your diet by sneaking in unnecessary calories.

6. Don't stress out. Stress increases the hormone cortisol, which lowers testosterone and causes you to store fat instead of burning it.

7. Sleep well. Studies have shown that sleep-deprived people have slower metabolisms and higher levels of cortisol.

If you're in a plateau, don't give up. This is a normal part of working out. Resist the temptation to blow off your workout or pig out because "you're not seeing results." You'll only be spiting yourself. Hang in there. The results are on the way!!!!

Declare Your Independence From the Scale

The primary reason many women begin an exercise program is to reduce body weight. When translated into its visual equal, they're saying they want to lose inches or dress sizes.

It's not uncommon for an exerciser to lose fat weight and gain muscle weight without any change in total body weight on the scale. So, are you really any closer to your goals if you've lost inches but little or no weight? Absolutely!!

Strength training decreases stored body fat and replaces it with lean muscle mass. Lean muscle mass is actually smaller in size than an equal amount of body fat. Here is a visual example: Picture a small stone, which will represent lean muscle mass. The stone probably weighs 2 ounces. Now picture cotton balls, which in this case will represent body fat. How many cotton balls would it take to weigh 2 ounces? It would take many cotton balls to equal 2 ounces. Those cotton balls take up much more space that the stone, which is what body fat does. It takes up more space and pads your body while lean muscle mass is denser and gives a much more sculpted appearance.

In our mid-twenties we begin to lose lean muscle mass as part of the normal aging process. This process speeds up as we age and can accelerate up to a 1 pound loss of lean

The Mind-Body Connection

THE POWER OF POSITIVE THINKING

Think of yourself as healthy and fit. When your willpower starts to wane, bring up those images and don't let them go.

muscle mass each year. Here is why this is so significant. As you lose lean muscle, your metabolism slows down. One pound of lean muscle burns up to approximately 50 calories per day at rest, while one pound of body fat only burns about 5 calories per day at rest. Think about that. As you replace the lost lean muscle mass you will be speeding up your metabolism and burning more calories 24/7. Performing strength-training exercises is the only way to add lean muscle mass back onto your body.

Since lean muscle mass is also what enhances your physical appearance, committing to a long-term plan of strength training is critical to achieving and maintaining the well-toned yet very feminine look that so many women strive for.

So next time you hop on the scale, remember that the amount you weigh is not as important as the how much body fat you are storing, which is something that a scale can't tell you.

If you really want to measure just how you're body is changing, break out the tape measurer or try slipping into those jeans that you haven't been able to wear.

Develop a Positive Self-Image

Work to improve your self-image by avoiding self-defeating language. Don't put yourself down when talking to others, including your family and friends.

Check your body language. Slumped shoulders, fidgeting hands and feet, chewed-off fingernails, arms crossed in front of your chest, and downcast eyes may indicate to others that you are insecure. Instead, make a conscious effort to appear confident. Make eye contact when talking to others.

Encourage yourself by recognizing your strengths and good qualities while never expecting yourself to be perfect.

Keep It Balanced

Contributed by Susan Scholl
www.LifeBalancingForWomen.com

Allow your fitness program to comfortably fit into your life rather than forcing it. This is accomplished by keeping balance between all the important components of your life. You will find that your fitness program can naturally blend into your daily activities. Your fitness program is not meant to rule your life but rather to compliment who you are and the lifestyle by which you live. As you work toward making your fitness program part of your routine, you will find that it can feel just as natural to work out as it is to get a good night's rest.

It's important to know that fitness is a course of action that takes place over a lifetime. Not only is it important to get off to a good start, but also maintaining your fitness program over the years will provide you with so many benefits. It's easy to get caught up in the excitement of starting something new and end up

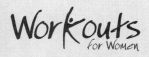

putting too much effort into the startup phase rather than keeping it in balance with the rest of your life. Start slowly with reasonable expectations. Results will come over a period of time and will last for years when you take good care of yourself and set realistic goals. Change happens gradually so be patient with yourself and go at a reasonable pace.

During the course of designing your fitness activities, set reasonable goals so you will continue to be encouraged as you work toward them. For example, if you try to exercise strenuously for 7 days a week with no rest, you risk burnout and disappointment. This is a lifetime commitment, so concentrate on incorporating fitness into your daily life. Try to keep other aspects of your life in balance—spirituality, family and friends, education, career, and just plain fun and relaxation. Perhaps you can even recruit a family member or a friend to become involved in physical activity with you. What better way to bond with someone than to take an hour walk through nature together?

As you develop a healthy fitness schedule, take small steps by easing into exercise and eating properly. Approach this with the goal of making some positive life changes for yourself rather than an a "fad" in your life that will only last for a limited period of time. You can incorporate some new healthy recipes into your food preparation a little at a time rather than making drastic changes. Try some new "mini-meals." These are meals you can spread out through the day by eating five or six small meals rather than three large ones. Incorporate fitness into your new life-style with fun leisure activities such as biking, playing tennis or golf, or walking. Each season of the year brings its own beauty to nature. Balance your outdoor activities so you enjoy the change of seasons.

By example and family participation, you can teach your children to eat healthy and remain fit as a lifestyle. What they learn now will stay with them throughout their lives.

Watch your progress by keeping a journal. Concentrate on keeping in balance and avoid becoming discouraged by looking at what you have accomplished. Be realistic in goal-setting and don't overdo activities in any one area of your life. It's critical to find a balance between family and friends, work and chores, and self-care. Your journal will give you lots of clues over a period of time on where you succeed and where you can focus more positive energy.

By enjoying fitness as part of your healthy lifestyle along with balancing other important elements of your life, you will be a whole, healthy woman. You will find that your self-esteem is greatly increased along with your energy. Have fun with it. Enjoy your new lifestyle of fitness and balance.

The Mind-Body Connection

APPENDIX I
Workout Log

Use this Workout Log to track your weekly workouts and keep you focused.

Recommended Exercise Schedules

Weight Loss. To lose weight, a combination of Aerobic workouts and Circuit workouts works the best. Suggested Circuit schedule is to complete 3 to 5 Circuit workouts each week. If you are a beginner, start with 1 or 2 circuits per day working up to four Circuits per day as your fitness level increases. Circuit training will burn calories during the activity and more importantly will build lean muscle mass, which will increase your metabolism 24/7 which is key to long term weight control. Also suggested is at least two 20 to 30 minute Aerobic sessions each week to burn additional calories and expedite weight loss. Aerobic sessions may be completed on the same days as the Circuit sessions or on alternate days if your schedule dictates. Always allow at least one rest day each week.

Shaping and Toning. If you are at your ideal weight and do not struggle with weight control but would like to firm up and re-shape your physique, the suggested schedule is to complete 3 to 5 Circuit workouts per week. If you are a beginner, start with 1 or 2 circuits per day, working up to 4 Circuits per day as your fitness level increases. It's safe to Circuit Train on consecutive days if your scheduling dictates. Since Circuit Training uses lower weight and higher repetitions to fatigue the muscles, the result is a well-sculpted lean look rather than bulk. Always allow at least one rest day each week.

Maintenance Programs

Weight Control. Once you have reached your fitness goals, if weight control is a challenge for you, choose this maintenance program. Commit to a lifestyle of fitness by scheduling in time for 2 to 3 Circuit workouts per week consisting of 3 or 4 Circuit rotations per workout and 2 Aerobic workouts 20 to 30 minute each week. Always allow at least one rest day each week.

Workouts for Women

Shape Control. Once you have reached your fitness goals, if weight control is not a challenge for you but you want to maintain your firmness and muscle tone then choose this maintenance program. Commit to a lifestyle of fitness by scheduling in time for 3 to 4 workouts per week consisting of 3 or 4 Circuit rotations per workout. Always allow at least one rest day each week.

Instructions

In the Circuit row, log how many Circuit rotations you've completed. In the Cardio row, log how many minutes you spent doing cardiovascular activities such as walking, biking, jumping rope or any other cardiovascular activity of your choice.

SAMPLE WORKOUT LOG

Start Date: _____ End Date: _____

WEEK		SUNDAY	MONDAY	TUESDAY	WEDNESDAY	THURSDAY	FRIDAY	SATURDAY	TOTAL
1	Circuits		3 Circuits				4 Circuits		
	Cardio			30 min. Stationary bike		30 min. Stationary bike			
2	Circuits	4 Circuits	4 Circuits						
	Cardio			30 min. Stationary bike		30 min. Stationary bike			
3	Circuits		3 Circuits		3 Circuits		3 Circuits		
	Cardio			30 min. Stationary bike		30 min. Stationary bike			

WORKOUT LOG

Start Date: _____ End Date: _____

WEEK		SUNDAY	MONDAY	TUESDAY	WEDNESDAY	THURSDAY	FRIDAY	SATURDAY	TOTAL
1	Circuits								
	Cardio								
2	Circuits								
	Cardio								
3	Circuits								
	Cardio								
4	Circuits								
	Cardio								
5	Circuits								
	Cardio								
6	Circuits								
	Cardio								
7	Circuits								
	Cardio								
8	Circuits								
	Cardio								

Workouts for Women

APPENDIX II
Food Journal

For optimal success, monitor your food consumption by keeping a visual record. Use the Food Journal to record the time you eat, what you eat and the activity that you were doing while you ate. It's also very helpful to track your mood at the time you were eating. This enables you to observe patterns in how activities and moods affect your food choices. Once you pinpoint what is negatively effecting your food choices you can work on making the appropriate changes.

For instance, perhaps you have a tendency to snack on crackers or cookies in the early evening while watching TV. With that knowledge, you can now plan to have a healthier alternative snack on hand for that time of the day since you know that is normally your prime snacking time. Another possible solution is to do something different during that time of the day to break the habit such as taking a walk or reading a book in a different room instead of sitting where you normally do to snack.

SAMPLE FOOD JOURNAL

Day/Time	Food	Activity
3/25 7am	Egg and cheese with bagel, hot tea	Breakfast watching news, relaxed
11am	1/4 cup trail mix	Relaxed, working at desk
1pm	Turkey and Swiss cheese wrap, grapes	Relaxed, at kitchen table
4pm	1 cup Bean Soup, 4 whole wheat crackers	A little nervous, thinking about job interview later this week
6:45pm	Chicken Cordon Blu and salad	Tired, long day
9:30pm	Graham crackers ... too many!	Watching TV, bored, lonely
3/26 6am	Cheerios and 1/2 cup yogurt	Breakfast watching news, relaxed
12:pm	Two Taco Bell Burritos	Driving, rushing to meeting
8pm	TV dinner and bowl of ice cream	Tired!
10pm	Vanilla Wafers and milk	Watching news, tired!
3/27 6am	Fruit and Yogurt	Relaxed, day off today
12:30pm	Chicken Caesar Salad	Lunch out with friend, shopping day at the mall, relaxed
6:30pm	Two Slices cheese Pizza	Food court, with friend at the mall, tired
3/28 6am	Yogurt and fruit	Nervous about interview tomorow.
11am	1/4 cup trail mix	Relaxed, eating at desk while working
1pm	Tuna Salad sandwich, grapes	Relaxed, lunch break
6:30pm	Salmon and sweet potato, salad	Relaxed
9:30pm	Graham crackers ... too many again.	Nervous about interview tomorow.

OOD JOURNAL

y/Time	Food	Activity

Special Book Buyers Discount
for purchases at www.WorkoutsForWomen.com
Enter this exclusive Book Buyer's Discount Code during checkout and Receive **25%** off your first purchase at www.WorkoutsForWomen.com.

DISCOUNT CODE: Book0105

Visit www.WorkoutsForWomen.com for our complete list of products including fitness equipment, online personal training, videos, meal plans, and quality skin care products.

Workouts For Women Circuit Shaping DVD or VHS
Complete workout video of all 10 circuits included in this book.
Bursting with over 90 different exercises, these 10 total-body, circuit shaping routines can each be completed in less than 12 minutes. This is ideal if you are short on time or just getting back into exercise. For a longer and more challenging workout, simply choose complete 2, 3, or 4 circuits for up to a 48-minute workout. Follow along for one-on-one instructions from your trainer, Joni.

Personal Training with Our Achievers Club
Don't go it alone!
Receive guidance and support from the Leaders in Women's Fitness. We are here to support, coach, even challenge you to achieve your goals.
- Personal Training: New Circuit Training Workouts online each week with an Accountability System to keep you on track.
- Community Support System from women just like you who have become Achievers.

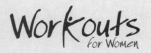

JAN 0 7 2005